COMMUNITY MEDICINE: A TEXTBOOK
FOR NURSES AND HEALTH VISITORS

Community Medicine
A Textbook for Nurses and Health Visitors

W.E. WATERS, MB BS, DIH, FFCM
Professor of Community Medicine

K.S. CLIFF, DM, MB BS, MRCS, LRCP, DPH, FFCM
Senior Lecturer in Community Medicine

University of Southampton. Honorary Specialists in Community Medicine,
Wessex Regional Health Authority.

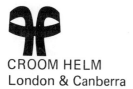

CROOM HELM
London & Canberra

Croom Helm Ltd, Provident House, Burrell Row,
Beckenham, Kent BR3 1AT

British Library Cataloguing in Publication Data

Waters, W.E.
   Community medicine
   1. Community health nursing — Great Britain
   I. Title.   II. Cliff, K.S.
   362.1'0425   RT98

   ISBN 0-7099-2751-7

Printed and bound in Great Britain
by Billing and Sons Ltd, Worcester.

CONTENTS

PREFACE

In this book we wish to introduce members of the nursing profession, and in particular those concerned with caring for people in the community, to the concepts of community medicine and the science upon which it is based, namely epidemiology. More and more our nursing colleagues are becoming involved in the management of health services, either as members of teams or in their own right. They need, as do doctors and administrators, to understand the distribution of disease in the community in which they work, or for which they have responsibility, and what effects and alters the pattern of disease in order to plan for, and evaluate the outcome of, the services they are providing.

No longer is it acceptable to adopt the authoritarian approach that what was done before must be correct. Technology has changed medical care, and hence the nurse's role, requiring increased skills and demands upon those skills. We suggest, however, that whilst nurses should be equipped not only with these increased practical skills of nursing patients, they should also be equipped to take a broader view of their work, to ask questions about the patients they see and the care given in epidemiological terms, that is: what is the distribution of the disease in the community which they see and what is the cause?

In compiling this book we have drawn upon a series of articles which we were asked to furnish for the *Nursing Mirror* and we wish to acknowledge the Editor and his staff's help with these original articles. We also wish to acknowledge the kind permission of Blackwell Scientific Publications Ltd to reproduce Figure 2.1, Churchill Livingstone to reproduce Table 2.2, the Editor of the *British Journal of Preventive and Social Medicine* to reproduce Figure 4.1, the Editor of *The Lancet* to reproduce Figures 7.1 and 7.2, and to the National and Local Government Officers' Association to draw upon material first prepared for their NALGO correspondence course. We express our thanks also to Miss Margery Dancer, Senior Community Nurse Tutor, Knowle Hospital, and her colleagues, and to Miss P. Gastrell, Lecturer in Health Visiting, for their comments on the original articles for the *Nursing Mirror*. Finally to our secretary, Wendy Couper, for typing the many drafts of the manuscript and tables.

1 INTRODUCTION TO THE HISTORY AND DEVELOPMENT OF COMMUNITY MEDICINE

The term 'community medicine' was first used to describe a specific area of work in medical care in the 'Report of the Royal Commission on Medical Education' (1968: 66-70). This report outlined the function of community medicine as being as follows:

A specialty practised by epidemiologists and administrators of medical services — e.g. medical officers of local authorities, central health or other government departments, hospital boards or industry — and by the staffs of corresponding academic departments. It is concerned not with the treatment of individual patients but with the broad questions of health and disease, in for example, particular geographical and occupational sections of the community and the community at large . . . It embraces many activities and interests and includes doctors employed in different spheres, partly because the health services have developed in this country several different authorities.

The report indicated that, whilst community medicine made use of a variety of skills and techniques (epidemiology and statistics), these were not exclusive to community medicine. Doctors working in community medicine did not have a monopoly of responsibility or of contribution and many other people's skills were required in the process of caring.

In 1972 the Faculty of Community Medicine was established in association with the Royal Colleges of Physicians of the United Kingdom to bring together those doctors who were practising within the broad definition of community medicine. At that time this group included doctors working in local health authorities, regional hospital boards, Department of Health and Social Security and academic departments. The Faculty of Community Medicine laid down guidelines for the admission of doctors to the new specialty as 'foundation members', but since 1976 entry has been by examination and training programmes have been established for doctors seeking a career in community medicine. Since 1974 appropriately qualified doctors working in community medicine within the National Health Service are appointed as specialists, equating with clinical specialists (consultants). Within community medicine there are now two senior specialist grades, Regional Medical Officer and District Medical Officer. These posts are principally administrative in function and the holders are respectively members of Regional and District Management Teams of Officers.

The Faculty of Community Medicine also accepted within its membership those doctors who were then working in the local authority preventive health services who did not wish to become specialists. These doctors practised preventive medicine under the generic title of Community Clinical Medical Officers and are co-ordinated by the District Medical Officers of the District Health Authorities. The principal function of this group of doctors lies in the practice of clinical preventive medicine through the child health, school health, vaccination and immunisation and, increasingly, occupational and adult preventive health services. This area of community medicine is termed Community Health.

Community medicine, as practised by specialists, is concerned with the following activities: the promotion of health and the prevention of disease, with the assessment of a community's health needs and with the provision of services to communities in general and to special groups within them. It complements the concern of clinical medicine with the help of individual patients. Epidemiology is the science fundamental to the study and practice of community medicine (*Community Medicine* 1982: 49).

Early Developments 1800-1849

Concern about the health of the population in England and Wales came as a consequence of the industrial revolution, which had begun in the eighteenth century. The social and health aspects related to the changes associated with this pattern of development were not immediately recognised. With the development of industries economic change occurred in the country and there was a move away from the predominantly agricultural economy to an industrially based one. This industrial growth required labour to work in factories and mills and led to an expansion of existing towns and cities. This expansion brought new major social and health problems, principally related to the environment. Housing had to be provided for the workers but was often of poor standard, unplanned and built close to the places of employment, thus being subject to industrial atmospheric pollution. Water supplies and sewage disposal systems were often totally inadequate and drinking water was often drawn from polluted sources. Evidence suggested that despite the poor social conditions in many towns and developing cities, there had been, since 1700, a gradual increase in the population of England and Wales. This increase continued through the nineteenth century as shown by decennial national censuses instituted in 1801, when the population was approximately nine million (McKeown and Lowe 1977: 5). This growth in the population, shown in Figure 1.1, has been considered to be due principally to a decline in overall mortality, linked with improved nutrition. Peasant agriculture was gradually changed to more modern farming methods during the agricultural revolution, which preceded and partly led to the industrial revolution. As mechanisation became available further improvement in farming followed and improved nutrition was, therefore, linked to an increase in the actual amount of land being cultivated as well as the type of foods grown. By the middle of the nineteenth century increased trading with other countries also made cheap food imports available to the population, helping to supplement home-grown produce (McKeown and Lowe 1977: 19-20).

Figure 1.1: England and Wales: Enumerated Population 1801-1981

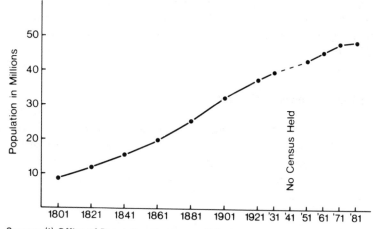

Source: (i) Office of Population Censuses and Surveys, Part II, Table Populations (1971), (HMSO London 1972) p. 2. (ii) Office of Population Censuses and Surveys, Preliminary Report Census 1981 (HMSO, London, 1982), p. 5.

Much of the ill-health in England and Wales during this period stemmed from infectious diseases, such as typhoid, tuberculosis, dysentery, scarlet fever and smallpox. In addition, there was a risk of importation of other infectious diseases, including cholera and yellow fever (neither of which were endemic in Britain), due to the increased trading with other countries. It was the fear of the importation of yellow fever into England and Wales at the beginning of the nineteenth century which was to lead to the establishment, in 1805, of what was in effect the first public health advisory committee, in the form of the Central Board of Health. The Board, which was to remain operational for only one year, consisted of both lay and medical advisers. The Board's most notable achievements were the defining of the principles and practices for the management of infectious disease, not only in relation to yellow fever but also other infectious diseases such as plague and smallpox. The Board's influence was, however, perpetuated through proposals put forward in relation to the control of smallpox and in 1809 the first Vaccination Board was established with the objective of promoting vaccination against smallpox as a means of protection and prevention of this disease within the population.

This period also witnessed two notable pieces of legislation which, when brought together, formed the basis for the development of medical statistics and epidemiology. These were The Population Act 1800 and the Registration of Births, Marriages and Deaths Act 1836.

Population Act 1800

The introduction of the Population Act stemmed from the central government's lack of information about the growth in population and hence the requirement for the provision of resources. An attempt had been made to enumerate the population in England and Wales through a Bill introduced in 1753, but this had lapsed. With the growth of the industrial revolution and population mobility, central government became concerned that they knew little about the total population or the changes that were occurring. The first census of the population in England and Wales under the Population Act was held in 1801. Subsequently a national census has been held every ten years (when the year ends in a one) with the exception of 1941. Initially the census data were co-ordinated by a government department but in 1841 the administration of the census became part of the responsibility of the General Register Officer controlled by the Registrar General, this post being created in 1836.

Births, Marriages and Deaths Act 1836

In 1836 two Acts were introduced, the Births and Deaths Registration Act and the Marriages Act and these were combined into one Act which became operative on 1 July 1837. This Act initially required only voluntary registration of births, marriages and deaths and this information became termed 'vital statistics'. The Act provided facilities for registration through a Registrar of Births, Marriages and Deaths, based on geographic areas formed by boundaries of 'Poor Law Units', which generally covered a number of parishes. The returns were passed by the Registrar to the General Register Office in London. In due course the geographic areas covered by the Registrars were extended (but were still based upon parishes) to form registration districts. Compulsory registration came into force in 1874 and subsequently there have been minor changes to the original Act, but in essence since 1 July 1837 a complete record of births, marriages and deaths has been available in this country.

The office of Registrar General, created in 1836, carried with it responsibility for the General Register Office, combining in 1841 census data with registration data of births, marriages and deaths. This was to continue in operation until 1970 when the General Register Office was combined with the Government Social Survey to form the Office of Population Censuses and Surveys; the post of Registrar General being maintained (Office of Population Censuses and Surveys 1980: 1).

At the time of the establishment of the General Register Office, a post of Medical Adviser was created and Dr William Farr was appointed the first Medical Adviser. Using the information available to him, Dr Farr was able to develop the basis of modern epidemiological and statistical investigations, using the census data combined with the registration data. Dr Farr also developed his own system of classifying mortality data and had sought, at an early stage after the introduction of the Births, Marriages and Deaths Act, the co-operation of the medical profession in identifying the cause of death on the death certificate. This data was, therefore, to provide him with vital information about mortality in England and Wales. The combination of the census and vital statistics data also allowed Dr Farr to develop the system of producing life tables, that is estimating the life expectancy of the population at various ages, and the use of this will be considered in Chapter 2.

The value of mortality data and population statistics was highlighted by Dr Farr in demonstrating, subsequent to the 1853-4 London cholera outbreak, that this disease was probably water-borne, and thus was able to support the hypothesis of Dr John Snow that deaths from cholera were linked to polluted water supplies (Office of Population Censuses and Surveys 1980: 4).

This period was also to see the first milestones in the development of community medicine, with the introduction of the Public Health Act 1848. This piece of legislation was in a large part due to the work of Edwin Chadwick, a social reformer of that period, who undertook a study of conditions within the working population and published a report in 1842 entitled *The sanitary conditions of the labouring classes*. In this report he demonstrated, with the help of a colleague, Dr John Southwood, and using data from the General Register Office, that the life expectancy of labourers in England and Wales was only 20 years, compared to 45 years for the gentry. Dr Farr, using data from the Registrar General's Office, was also able to demonstrate differences in mortality between the populations of towns and cities compared to counties. In his report to the Registrar General in 1839 he indicated that the crude death rate for people living in towns and cities was 1370 per 100,000 compared to 857 per 100,000 for the counties. The causes of death were based on Farr's own classification, which was to remain in operation until 1900 when the international list of causes of deaths was adopted (Office of Population Censuses and Surveys 1980: 24).

Chadwick's report and analyses by Dr Farr were to have profound effects on the social conscience of the government. Chadwick proposed that improvements in water supply, removal of house refuse, proper drainage and street cleansing were fundamental to the problem of the ill-health in the population. The Public Health Act 1848 established a General Board of Health (Central Government) and Local Boards of Health (Local Authorities). It was unfortunate, however, that no government minister was appointed to take responsibility for the General Board of Health, so that much of the Act's impetus was to be lost. Though the Act empowered Local Boards of Health to appoint medical officers of health with responsibility for environmental conditions and infectious disease, the response was slow. The Act did not apply to London and did not apply to those towns or cities which had invoked their own Acts of Parliament. The first medical officer of health was in fact appointed in 1847 in the City of Liverpool under a private Act of Parliament and by 1850 200 Local Boards of Health were established, of which 33 had appointed medical officers of health (Brockington 1965: 32-3).

In addition to medical officers of health, central government also had medical advisers to the General Board of Health and, thus, the 1848 Public Health Act created two of the precursor groups of doctors who were to form the future Faculty of Community Medicine. Doctors working at the General Board of Health were specifically involved in an administrative capacity and formed the precursor Civil Service Medical Officers. This period, therefore, saw the beginnings of the development of a public health service, the development of medical statistics and epidemiology through the work of Dr William Farr linked with the legislation on births, marriages and deaths and the census, social reforms allied to health through housing and improvement in working conditions. These changes and developments were to become part of the work of practitioners in community medicine.

1850-1899

This period was to see further growth in preventive legislation concerned with the public health of the community. The 1848 Public Health Act had tried to promote preventive legislation but had no central government direction. Between 1850 and 1870 a number of amendments were made to the 1848 Act and new legislation was introduced in 1868 and 1870 through the 'Sanitary Acts'. The 1868 Act facilitated and co-ordinated the existing legislation whilst the 1870 Act gave wide powers to local authorities in respect of the provision of sanitation, water supply, smoke and nuisance abatement as well as disease prevention.

Further legislation under the Local Government Board Act 1871 established a Local Government Board at central government level with a minister responsible for co-ordinating 'Health and Poor Law Duties'. This was followed, in 1872, by a further Public Health Act which defined and mapped the urban and rural sanitary authorities, making it compulsory for these authorities to appoint a medical officer of health, and the Public Health Act of 1875 laid down regulations relating to the range and duties of sanitary authorities and their medical officers of health.

The duties of the medical officer of health included environmental health, provision of fever hospitals, control of housing standards and food inspection, and the Act provided the basic legislation for public health which was to remain operative until the introduction of the National Health Service in 1948. Further legislation under a Local Government Act of 1888 was to establish county borough and county councils and enable the latter to appoint their own medical officers of health. Under this Act, doctors appointed on a full-time basis to counties or district health authorities with populations of over 50,000 had to have a recognised qualification, namely the Diploma in Public Health. The Diploma in Public Health became registerable with the General Medical Council in 1886, and thus community medicine specialists of that period were defined by this specialist qualification. The first Diploma in Public Health in the British Isles was instituted in 1870 by Trinity College, Dublin, and in the UK by the University of Cambridge in 1875 (Frazer 1950: 229-30).

This period also saw the development of a multidisciplinary approach to community medicine. Dr Thomas Turner, in Manchester, drew attention to the high infant mortality rate and in particular the high perinatal and neonatal mortality (deaths in the first week, including stillbirths and first month of life respectively) amongst the uneducated mothers living in the poorer areas of the cities. In 1862 the Manchester and Salford Ladies Health Society was established, undertaking visiting mothers with newborn babies as soon as possible after delivery to give advice on simple hygiene. These women were to be the forerunners of the modern health visitors and the Society was recognised by the City of Manchester who came to an arrangement such that a proportion of the salaries of the Health Society were paid for by the Authority (Baly 1973: 61).

Florence Nightingale, whose interest in nursing extended also to the prevention of disease, drew attention to the appalling lack of simple basic knowledge of hygiene in the population in her 'Notes on Nursing 1858' (Brockington 1965: 34). In these notes she outlined some of the reasons for child mortality stating: 'Women, and the best of women, are woefully deficient in sanitary knowledge; although it is to women that we must look first and last for its application as far as household hygiene is concerned. The causes of the enormous child mortality are perfectly well known; they are chiefly want of cleanliness, want of ventilation, careless dieting and clothing, want of white-washing, in one word, defective household hygiene.' In the latter part of her life, Florence Nightingale was to contribute further to the development of health education and health visiting, making use of the Local Government Act of 1881 which gave county councils the power to spend money on technical education. In 1891 she wrote to the chairman of the Technical Instruction Committee of her county (Buckinghamshire) requesting funding for lady health visitors to receive instruction, which was classified as technical education. A special course of training was started and a number of other counties were to follow the example, but the main thrust of health visiting was to develop later (Brockington 1965: 43).

Another group of nurses working in the community were those involved in midwifery and moves had been made to register midwives through the Obstetrical Society, founded during the 1860s. The Society became responsible for certifying midwives and the first certificates were issued in 1872. By 1899 5,000 midwives were to hold the certificate. During this period also general nursing had been developed through the efforts of Miss Nightingale and the first school of nursing was opened

at St Thomas's Hospital in July 1860. This early beginning was to lead
to a development of nursing schools in both Voluntary and Poor Law
hospitals, but in the latter strong resistance was met by many boards of
guardians, as they saw this as an increased demand on the rates. Despite
all these activities, both in the field of general nursing, midwifery and
early health visiting, some aspects of the health of the population were
to be found wanting.

1900-1948

This period was to see an expansion of the influence of community
medicine from that purely relating to environmental health and infectious disease control into areas of personal preventive health provision,
and the administration of hospitals. In terms of the developments of
the provision of personal health services, these were to develop in two
main areas:
(1)   The provision of a school health service
(2)   The provision of a maternity and child health service.

School Health Services

At the very beginning of this period, 1901-2, ill-health in England and
Wales was brought to the forefront of debate by the finding that some
40 per cent of young men presenting for recruitment to serve in the
British Army in South Africa were medically unfit. The major defects
leading to rejection were want of physical development, defective vision,
diseases of the heart and bad dentition. Some of these conditions
reflected general poor nutrition among the labouring classes, who at
that time proportionately formed a larger group of the population than
today. In response to these findings the government established the
Inter-departmental Committee on Physical Deterioration 1903 which
was to report in 1904. Included in the recommendations of the report
were; the introduction of systematic medical inspections of children at
school, to be imposed as a statutory duty on every school authority;
registration of stillbirths; anthropomorphic measurements of children;
education including the teaching of domestic science to girls; and training of mothers by health visitors in the care of infants (Essex-Cater
1967: 73).
    Of particular concern was the state of schoolchildren in England and
Wales who lived in large towns and cities and came from labouring
classes. Some local authorities had instituted free meals for needy

children and in other authorities voluntary associations had provided these. Central government was to act upon the inter-departmental report by passing two pieces of legislation, the Education Acts of 1906 and 1907.

Education (Provision of meals) Act 1906. This Act authorised local authorities to assist in the distribution of free meals to needy children by providing staff to help voluntary associations. Where voluntary associations were not in being or could not fulfil the whole of the task, local authorities were allowed to buy food for distribution. Progressive authorities, such as Liverpool, Manchester and London, immediately extended their existing voluntary schemes to provide free school meals for needy children. This Act provided the legal basis, therefore, for what, in some cases, had been occurring previously, in terms of providing for certain groups of the population.

Education (Administrative provisions) Act 1907. This Act established the School Health Service whereby all elementary schoolchildren were required to have *compulsory* periodic medical inspections. Two examinations were to be carried out; on entry to the elementary school and on leaving to proceed to secondary education. In addition, the Act allowed authorities to treat minor medical conditions, such as ringworm and head lice. At central government level the Act brought into being within the Board of Education a medical service and at local level medical officers of health became responsible for the School Health Service holding the joint appointment of medical officer of health and school medical officer. To support the doctors, health visitors and school nurses were to become integrated into the overall School Health Service and, in particular, health visitors therefore could liaise between the home and school. The Act of 1907 was to set the pattern in terms of examination of schoolchildren until 1948, though with minor amendments. These included an extension of school medical inspections from elementary into secondary school and the provision, in 1918, of open air schools. The main function of the School Medical Service was to maintain a healthy school population both within elementary and secondary schools.

Maternity and Child Health Services

A major concern had been the continuing high infant mortality rate in some parts of the country and health visiting had been recognised as of importance in reducing this mortality rate by early contact with mothers. This was confirmed by a study in Huddersfield in 1905 where, through the co-operation with Registrars of Births, Marriages and Deaths, the medical officer of health had been notified of all births registered in Huddersfield, allowing early contact by health visitors with the mothers. Based on this evidence, an Act was introduced in 1907 whereby notification of births by Registrars was to be provided on a voluntary basis to local health authorities. This became compulsory under the Notification of Birth (Extension) Act 1915 and this require- ment has continued to the present time, notification being made to district medical officers (Essex-Cater 1967: 73).

In the late nineteenth century, in addition to health visiting, some progressive authorities had introduced infant welfare clinics, milk depots and schools for mothers, all aimed at preventing the avoidable morbidity and mortality amongst infants. Infant mortality rates in 1906 ranged from 111 per 1,000 live births in Brighton to 212 per 1,000 in Burnley. The north and west showed higher mortality rates compared to the south and east in England and Wales but, despite these findings, legislation in respect of the provision of maternity and child welfare services was not enacted until 1918. The 1918 Maternity and Child Welfare Act allowed the establishment of health visiting services, infant welfare clinics and ante-natal clinics for expectant mothers (which pro- gressive authorities had already been providing). The development of these services was dependent upon recruitment of health visitors and, by 1918, some 3038 health visitors were employed in local health authorities in maternity and child welfare services as well as in the school health services. Initially health authorities laid down their own standards of training and qualification for health visitors, but in 1908 the Royal Sanitary Institute, later to become the Royal Society for the Promotion of Health, introduced an examination for health visitors and school nurses. In 1962 the Training Council for Health Visitors became responsible for the formal training of health visitors and the work of this council and its development has been discussed by Wilkie (1979).

Further improvements in the personal health care services came with the establishment, under the Midwives Act 1902, of the Central Mid- wives Board. This Act required midwives to be registered and made the Central Midwives Board responsible for the training, certification and practice of the work of midwives. In 1918 a further Act enabled local authorities to help with the training of midwives, who at that time were still self-employed. This situation was to remain until 1936 when a salaried service was introduced for midwives and those not working in hospitals were employed in domiciliary midwifery services run by local authorities.

Hospital Services

The development of considerable importance was the formation in 1919 of the Ministry of Health, based on the old Central Board of Health. The medical staff of the Central Board transferred to the new Ministry and took responsibility for co-ordination and advice on aspects of health care, though the Poor Law administration, including their hospitals, were to remain outside government control. The chief medical officer to the Ministry of Health also held the joint appointment of chief medical adviser to the Board of Education, allowing for co-ordination of preventive services within the community, both adult and children. The provision of the Ministry of Health brought into being the Civil Service Medical Department, whose staff were to form one of the groups of doctors, some of whom were eventually to become community medicine specialists and members of the Faculty.

In 1929 a significant piece of legislation, namely the Local Government Act 1929, abolished the Poor Law system and passed the responsibility for the hospitals run by the Poor Law guardians to local authorities. In addition, this Act empowered local authorities to provide their own hospital facilities, and thus the medical officers of health were now involved not only in preventive services but also in the management of curative services. During this period the medical officers of health therefore wielded considerable power in terms of the provision of services for the community and this was to last until 1948, with the introduction of the National Health Service.

1948 Onwards

This period was to see the greatest change in the development of community medicine. The National Health Service, established in 1948 as a tripartite service covering hospital services, community services under the local authority and general practitioner services, introduced yet another group of doctors into community medicine. These were the administrative medical officers to the regional hospital boards, who were responsible for the organisation of hospital services. Medical officers of health lost control of hospitals in 1948 and reverted purely to environmental and personal preventive services, a role they had played from 1848 to 1929, when they also had control of some aspects of the hospital provision. This group of doctors were to lose further aspects of their work, namely social work in relation to mental handicap and mental illness, which in 1968 was to pass to the new social work departments of the county borough and county councils.

The reorganisation of the National Health Service in 1974 was to bring together the administration of the health services under regional and area health authorities, and it was this proposed reorganised structure which was paramount in drawing together those people practising in community medicine within a Faculty of Community Medicine in 1972. The Faculty was faced with the task of drawing together the expertise of four groups of doctors who could be identified as belonging to community medicine, under the definition in the report of the Royal Commission on Medical Education (1968: 66-70). These were:

(1)   Doctors working in local health authority services. These were the most numerous group and comprised county, county borough, municipal borough and rural district medical officers of health, and their supporting medical staff. The majority of these doctors held the Diploma in Public Health.

(2)   Doctors in the regional hospital boards. Many of these doctors had wide experience in the organisation and development of hospital services but did not necessarily possess a Diploma in Public Health, though some had higher clinical qualifications.

(3)   Doctors in the Civil Service Medical Department. This group of doctors again did not necessarily hold the Diploma in Public Health but many had been recruited from the hospital service and had a wide variety of higher medical, surgical and other professional qualifications.

(4)   Doctors working in academic departments. These were departments of public health, social medicine, social and preventive medicine, and basically provided the research influence based on epidemiological and statistical skills.

Together, these four groups formed the core of the new Faculty of Community Medicine and, as indicated earlier, the Faculty established criteria for entry as a member prior to the establishment of a proper examination.

The tripartite structure disappeared with the reorganisation of the National Health Service on 1 April 1974 and community medicine specialists were to take posts either at regional or area levels. In multi-district area health authorities some specialists became members of district management teams, which were geographical areas within an area health authority. These teams were responsible for the day-to-day organisation and management of services within a framework of policies established by the area health authority. This pattern was to continue until 1 April 1982 when area health authorities were abolished and district health authorities established. At this point the area medical officer posts and specialists in community medicine at area level were abolished and the new district medical officer posts, with their supporting specialists, were formed. Figure 1.2 identifies the development of community medicine from 1974 to 1982 and Figure 1.3 the present position, subsequent to the reorganisation on 1 April 1982.

Figure 1.2: Community Medicine Specialists: Structure in England and Wales 1 April 1974 to 31 March 1982

REGIONAL HEALTH AUTHORITY
_____

Regional Medical Officer
Co-ordinates the work of specialist colleagues

Specialist in Community Medicine

| Manpower Planning | Information and Epidemiology | Health Services Planning | Capital Planning (Hospitals, Health Centres) |

AREA HEALTH AUTHORITY
_____

(Single District)

Area Medical Officer
Co-ordinates the work of specialist colleagues

Specialists in Community Medicine

| Child Health | Social Services | Environmental Health | Planning and Information | Manpower (Teaching Authority only) |

Advise to Local Authorities

AREA HEALTH AUTHORITY
_____

(Multidistrict Area)

Area Medical Officer
Co-ordinates the work of specialist colleagues

Specialists in Community Medicine

Area office:

| Planning and Information | Social Services | Child Health | Manpower (Teaching Authority only) |

Advise to Local Authorities

District Offices: District Community Physicians
                    (Provided advice to Local Authority on
                    Environmental Health Matters: Proper Officer)

Figure 1.3: Community Medicine Specialists: Structure in England and Wales from 1 April 1982

REGIONAL HEALTH AUTHORITY

Regional Medical Officer
Co-ordinates the work of specialist colleagues

Specialists in Community Medicine

Manpower Planning	Information and Epidemiology	Health Services Planning	Capital Planning

DISTRICT HEALTH AUTHORITY

District Medical Officer
Co-ordinates the work of specialist colleagues

Specialists in Community Medicine
Duties will depend on the requirements of the District Health Authority but will include:

Planning and Information	Liaison with Local Authority	Environmental Health	Manpower Planning (Teaching Districts)

Community medicine today not only involves environmental and infectious disease control, but much wider aspects of health care such as planning, evaluation of services and the provision of information based on epidemiological studies. The basic principles of epidemiology and medical statistics remain the foundation stone of community medicine, as they have since its inception in the early nineteenth century. Whilst the emphasis may have changed from the control of infectious disease (though this is still an important aspect), to the prevention and planning of services for diseases found within modern society (e.g. accidents, chronic disabling diseases, heart disease) there remains a need for close co-operation between community medicine and other professions, particularly nursing.

Conversely, nurses must be able to appreciate the basis of community medicine, that is epidemiology and statistics, if they are also to be able to play a full part in health care planning, evaluation and particularly in prevention. Nurses have been taking a major role in determining health care policy, particularly since 1974 when they began to play an active part in management as members of regional, area and district management teams, as well as members of health care planning teams, which were established under the reorganised National Health Service in many of the area and district health authorities. Thus, there has been a changing pattern in the role which nurses have played, from purely a traditional one of nursing skills with limited administration relating only to nurses, to a broader one relating to health care services.

2

THE CHANGING PATTERN OF DISEASE
IN THE COMMUNITY FROM 1800

Introduction

This chapter will outline some of the major factors which have been identified as having particular influences on the changes in patterns of disease in England and Wales since 1800. Measurement of the changes in disease pattern can be obtained from two principal sources: morbidity (ill-health) and mortality (death). Chapter 1 outlined two major important pieces of legislation which have allowed epidemiologists to study changing patterns of disease in the community. These were The Population Act 1800 and The Births, Marriages and Deaths Act 1836. These Acts provided the essential tools for the epidemiologist to examine, in particular, mortality data in relation to the population, as well as examining the population changes by age groups and sex.

Morbidity data have proved more difficult to collect and early and subsequent studies have very often been related to specific populations and diseases. Florence Nightingale was one of the early epidemiologists and carried out studies into the morbidity and mortality amongst soldiers living in barracks, illustrating the high mortality amongst young men (Seymer 1957: 84-5). An example of a local morbidity study was that carried out by Pickles (1932: 31-2) into Sonne dysentery in Wensleydale, where he was the local general practitioner. Morbidity data was to become more readily available following the introduction of the National Health Service, and a number of routine morbidity data collection systems were introduced, particularly in respect of the hospital services. These have included the Hospital In-patient Inquiry, based on a one in ten sample of every discharge from (or death in) a National Health Service hospital in England and Wales since 1958, but excluding psychiatric hospitals which developed their own system, the Mental Health Inquiry, in 1964. A further system for collecting morbidity data based on hospital information was introduced in 1965 and termed the Hospital Activity Analysis. This system collected information on every discharge or death occurring in a National Health Service hospital, with the exception of obstetric and psychiatric hospitals. This system has been fully described in a book by Brewer and Rowe (1972).

Hospital data, as a source of morbidity data, are however limited in that they are not representative necessarily of the total morbidity within the population as a whole. For some conditions, for example acute renal failure, all people will be admitted to hospital for treatment, but for conditions such as chronic bronchitis, many patients will be treated at home by the general practitioner. Morbidity data have been collected by the Royal College of General Practitioners and by a number of individual general practitioners within their own practice (Morrel, Gage and Robinson 1970: 331-41).

Whilst mortality and morbidity data can indicate changes in the pattern of disease, the epidemiologist is concerned not only with the distribution over time of the disease within the population and how this has changed, but the determinants. From a study of the period a number of factors have been identified which are relevant to the change in pattern of disease in England and Wales since 1800. These include the determination of the cause of disease, social changes, population structure changes, changes in life style and an understanding of the relationship between occupation and disease. These factors will be discussed separately to illustrate their effect on the change in pattern of disease in England and Wales.

Determination of the Cause of Disease

The predominant diseases of the early and middle part of the nineteenth century were infectious in type. These included tuberculosis, scarlet fever and imported infectious diseases, for example cholera. Outbreaks of this latter disease occurred in England and Wales in 1831, 1848, 1853 and 1865. In 1848 an estimate was made that some 53,000 deaths were attributable to this cause and 19,000 deaths to diarrhoea (McKeown and Lowe 1977: 144). Observations of the possible mode of transmission of cholera were eventually to lead to its eradication. The observations and recording of cholera cases by Dr John Snow during the 1853-4 epidemic suggested a water-borne disease and that it was transmitted by the contamination of drinking water supplies from the excreta of patients with cholera.

The hypothesis that Dr Snow put forward was to be substantiated by Dr William Farr of the Registrar General's Office, working with a committee, who investigated the mortality from cholera in similar populations who were provided with water by two different water companies. Dr Farr was responsible for the analysis and he found that in 24,854 houses supplied by the Lambeth Company, serving a population of 166,906, there were 611 recorded cholera deaths during the 1853-4 outbreak. This gave a rate of 37 deaths per 10,000 of the population served. The Southwark and Vauxhall Company served a population of 268,171 and in the same period there were 3,476 cholera deaths, giving a rate of 130 deaths per 10,000 of the population served. This latter company was said to provide 'the filthiest stuff ever drunk by a civilised community'. The investigation suggested that deaths within the population served by the Southwark and Vauxhall Company were some three and a half times more common than those from the Lambeth Company. The committee further investigated cholera mortality in streets which were jointly supplied by the two companies and again found that the mortality amongst those houses provided by the Southwark and Vauxhall Company were three times as great as those from Lambeth (Frazer 1950: 63-4). These findings were to lead to the instigation of major engineering projects in London and other cities to provide a system of sewage disposal and the provision of clean safe drinking water supplies.

Other observations on the transmission of disease had identified overcrowding, malnutrition and poverty as factors associated with the spread of tuberculosis, which, in the early part of the nineteenth century, was a major cause of mortality and morbidity. A study of mortality data from tuberculosis was to show that this disease had begun to decline during the nineteenth and twentieth centuries even before the tubercle bacillus was identified by Koch or medical treatment became available, as shown in Figure 2.1. The introduction of specific therapy, coupled with the eradication of the tubercle bacillus from cattle were to act further in increasing the previous natural decline of the disease as a major cause of death.

The understanding of the cause of disease, through improved laboratory techniques coupled with diligent observations, was to lead to major developments in the control and treatment of many diseases, which were previously fatal. The discovery of penicillin and other antibiotics was to revolutionise the treatment of disease. Curative medicine came to the forefront and advances in surgery and other specialties increased the demand for care. This must be balanced, however, against the persistent epidemiological studies which were carried out to try and discover the causal factors of many of the diseases.

The work of Doll and Hill (1964: 1399-1410, 1460-7) on the associations between cigarette smoking, lung cancer and coronary heart disease, is a classic example of an epidemiological study into a modern problem. The study involved a ten year follow-up of British doctors and observations on the cause of death and their smoking habit. This study has probably had a major effect in producing a reduction in the proportion of people who smoke. During the period 1972 to 1980 (for

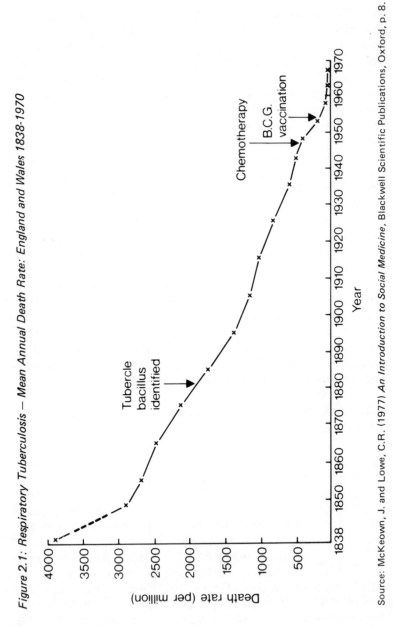

Figure 2.1: Respiratory Tuberculosis — Mean Annual Death Rate: England and Wales 1838-1970

Source: McKeown, J. and Lowe, C.R. (1977) An Introduction to Social Medicine, Blackwell Scientific Publications, Oxford, p. 8.

which figures are available) the proportion of men who smoked fell from 52 to 42 per cent, but only from 41 to 37 per cent in women (Social Trends 1982: 128). The determination of the cause of diseases and their subsequent control and/or eradication changes the pattern of disease within a population, because as the proportion of deaths from one disease declines, so the proportion contributed by the remainder increases and comes into greater prominence, although their total number may not actually increase. Changes in the cause of mortality in children provide an example of changing patterns of disease. During the period 1800 to 1900 infectious diseases were one of the most common causes of infant deaths. Since then not only has the number of deaths from infectious diseases decreased, but the pattern has altered.

Analysis of the cause of mortality amongst children aged 0-14 years, shown in Table 2.1, indicates how the pattern has changed in early life and with increasing age. Thus, by the age of 14 years accidents are a major contributing factor to childhood mortality. Change in disease pattern may alter the type of disease and its frequency because people survive longer and disease is associated with age and sex. Thus, an increasing longevity amongst the population will bring increased amounts of chronic disease. The pattern of disease has changed because of a number of factors, including eradication of infectious disease, improved social conditions (particularly nutrition), change in social habits, such as cigarette smoking, and increased life span. Thus, not all the changes have been medical; some have been social changes.

Table 2.1　England and Wales: Selected Causes of Death in Children Aged 0-14 Years per Million at Risk, 1978

Cause	< 1	1-4	5-9	10-14
Accidents	375.4	123.3	101.6	94.0
Congenital Abnormalities	3566.6	93.6	34.4	29.1
Respiratory Disease	1643.8	69.5	20.3	16.9
Malignant Disease	73.6	57.1	66.2	53.2

Source: Office of Population Censuses and Surveys, *Mortality Statistics by Cause, 1978* (England and Wales), Tables 1 and 2, pp. 1, 3-88.

Social Changes

Improvements in health and the decline in certain diseases had (as indicated in the previous section) begun to occur before the identification of the causal organisms of the disease or specific medical treatment. An understanding of the possible method by which disease was spread had enabled certain measures to be implemented and the work of Drs John

Snow and William Farr in respect of cholera (described in Chapter 1) provide an example. The early changes brought about by careful observation and epidemiological study of disease were primarily social. These included such aspects as improved housing, working conditions, pure safe water and sewage disposal.

The major reforms began in the early nineteenth century through the work of Edwin Chadwick. His work was to lead to the introduction of the 1848 Public Health Act and the subsequent legislation (referred to in Chapter 1). These pieces of legislation provided the framework for social reform with direct implications on health. Chadwick demonstrated a need for reform and social change through his careful studies of mortality in 553 urban districts in England and Wales during the period 1839-42. From an analysis of eight different districts within his total sample he indicated that the average life expectancy was related to social class and hence social conditions. Labourers (social class V) had a life expectancy of only 22 years, compared to 30 years for tradesmen (social class III), and 43 years for the gentry (social class I), which clearly showed a social class gradient (Cartwright 1977: 103).

In comparing mortality rates, as with comparing anything else, it is necessary to compare 'like with like'. One of the problems in comparing mortality rates for different social classes (or occupational groups, or any other populations) is that there may be different age structures in the groups being compared. As the chances of dying increase steeply with age it would not be appropriate to compare groups unless one took into account any age differences. Of course one could compare the mortality rate at specific ages, say, 45, 55 and 65 years, but the numbers in any one age group are relatively small and one would then be making several comparisons, not just one. This problem is usually tackled by using the standardised mortality ratio or SMR. This is the ratio, usually expressed as a percentage, of the number of deaths that actually occur in a population and the number of deaths expected, assuming that some standard rate has applied. A standardised mortality ratio of above 100 indicates a higher than average mortality experience and one below 100 indicates a lower than average mortality experience. The fact that it is standardised means that any differences in mortality are not due to differences in the ages of the populations.

Table 2.2 illustrates the differences in SMR for males aged 15-64 years, for different periods of time, by social class. For 1970-2 the SMR for social class I was 77, which indicates that they experienced only 77 per cent of the number of deaths that would have been expected had the national rates (for England and Wales) applied. Social classes

IV and V experienced 43 per cent and 37 per cent more deaths than expected, had the national rates applied. It will be clear that the figures in Table 2.2 compare the mortality experience for different social classes for four periods in time. The comparisons are based on the national death rates that occurred at those four periods of time. It is, therefore, not valid to directly compare the ratio for social class V in 1930-2 (111) with that of 1970-2 (137) and say that mortality rates have increased absolutely. The figures mean that whereas the mortality rate was 11 per cent more than the national rate of 1930-2, it was 37 per cent more than the national rate of 1970-2. But the national mortality rate for 1970-2 is considerably lower than that for 1930-2; it is the relative differences in mortality rates that have widened. This disturbing trend is only partially offset by the fact that there are now proportionately fewer people in social class V than there were 50 years ago, so the relative risks of dying have increased considerably in social class V but there is now a reduced proportion of people subjected to these risks.

Table 2.2: England and Wales: Standardised Mortality Ratios for Males Aged 15-64 Years for Four Selected Time Periods by Social Class

Social Class	1930-32	1949-53	1959-63	1970-72
I	90	86	76	77
II	94	92	81	81
III	97	101	100	104
IV	102	104	103	143
V	111	118	143	137
E & W	100	100	100	100

Note: The Standardised Mortality Ratio for England and Wales = 100.
Source: Barker, D.J.P. and Rose, C. (1979) *Epidemiology in Medical Practice*, Churchill Livingstone, Edinburgh, Table 4.2, p. 61.

The social class classification is based on a system used by the Registrar General whereby people with comparable qualifications and training are grouped together into what are termed social classes. This enables a very broad analysis to be made of occupational mortality with social classes. Examples of social class and occupation are shown in Table 2.3.

The major social policy changes which were to profoundly effect health were, as mentioned previously, related to engineering and housing, that is improving the environment. Housing was important and in

Table 2.3: Examples of Occupations by Social Class

Social Class	Occupations
I	Higher professional and administrative, e.g. lawyers, doctors, dentists
II	Other professional groups, employers in industry and retail trades, e.g. nurses, radiographers, managers
III N*	Skilled non-manual occupations, e.g. secretary, telephone operator
III M*	Skilled manual occupations, e.g. dental technicians
IV	Partly skilled occupations, e.g. hospital porter
V	Unskilled occupations, e.g. labourers, stevedores

*Because approximately half the population is in Social Class III it is divided into (N) non-manual and (M) manual.
Source: Office of Population Censuses and Surveys, *Classification of Occupations, 1980*, Appendix B2, pp. cv-cxvii.

1868 an Act (Torren's Act) made it a duty of house owners to keep their property in good repair. The 1875 Local Authority Act gave powers to local authorities to demolish and reconstitute blocks or areas of unsuitable and/or insanitary housing and this was followed in 1890 by the Housing of Working Classes Act which allowed local authorities to provide housing for the working classes. These initial Acts and subsequent legislation were to set the standards for housing and give wide powers to local authorities to improve the environment within which the people lived (Farrer-Brown and Warren 1965: 94-7).

Other social pressures were to bring about regulations in respect of child employment and hours of work and the recognition that social factors were important to health and these have been embodied in the World Health Organisation's definition of health, namely: 'A state of complete physical, mental and social well being'. The change in social factors has brought change in mortality and morbidity experience and has led to improved life expectancy and changes in the population structure.

Population Structure

The reduction in the number of deaths in childhood from infectious disease, particularly in the first year of life (infant mortality), coupled with improvements in social and welfare provision during the late nineteenth and early twentieth centuries led to changes in the life expectancy of the population, some of which are reflected in the present population structure.

This change in pattern was based on an increased expectation of life — the number of years on average an individual could expect to live at a given age. The most dramatic change has occurred in life expectancy at birth, as shown in Table 2.4. In 1901 life expectancy at birth was only 48.5 years for a male and 52.4 years for a female. In 1971 the comparable figures were 69 years and 75.3 years, a gain of approximately 22 years for both sexes. The table shows that women have a longer expectation of life compared to men, though one feature of the table is that the increase in life expectancy has not substantially altered for those aged 65 years and over. Thus, if people survived to 65 years in 1901 or 1971 they then experienced a similar mortality, as shown in Figure 2.2.

Table 2.4: England and Wales: Expectation of Life at Various Ages for Selected Years for Males and Females 1900-72

Age (Years)	1901-10	1930-32	1950-52	1970-72
Birth				
Male	48.5	58.7	66.4	69.0
Female	52.4	62.9	71.5	75.3
45 Years				
Male	23.3	25.5	26.5	27.4
Female	25.5	28.3	30.8	32.9
65 Years				
Male	10.8	11.3	11.7	12.2
Female	12.0	13.1	14.3	16.1

Source: Office of Population Censuses and Surveys, *Mortality Statistics 1978* (England and Wales), Table 22, p. 100.

Figure 1.1 in Chapter 1 showed the increase in the total population in England and Wales, though the rate of increase declined between 1971 and 1981 compared to the period 1961 to 1971. The main change in the population in recent years has been the high birth rate, particularly during the period 1960-70, followed by a steady decline and an increasing proportion of the population aged 65 years and over. This change in the population structure will become an increasingly important factor in the next 20 years, as the major change will be in the number of survivors in the age group 75 years and over. In 1901 there

*Figure 2.2. Sex and Age Structure of the Population (United Kingdom)
1901 and 1980*

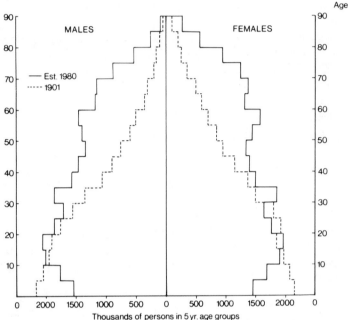

Thousands of persons in 5 yr. age groups

were approximately 1.7 million people aged 65 years and over, but by
1971 this had grown to 7.1 million, based on census data. The increasing proportion of elderly is expected to reach a peak in 1991, when
estimates suggest that approximately 8.3 million people will be aged 65
years and over (Carstairs 1981: 31-3).

The important aspect from the point of view of health care has been
in the proportional distribution of the elderly within the various age
groups. Disease in a population is associated with age and sex and with
increasing age the demand for health and social care becomes greater.
The important changes in the population distribution amongst those
aged 65 years and over is illustrated in Table 2.5, which indicates the
changes expected between 1978 and 1991, using 1978 as the baseline.
The table shows the increasing proportion of elderly aged 85 years and
over; the particular age group known to require a high level of support.
Changes in population structure particularly resulting in longevity produce changes in pattern of disease and, whilst not all disease requires
care in institutions, population changes must consider the marital status
of the elderly, that is whether there is a spouse to support a chronically

sick elderly partner in their own home. The age and health of the spouse are obviously important and in the older age groups spouses, even if alive, may not be able to look after chronically ill partners.

Table 2.5: Great Britain: Projected Elderly Population Aged 65 Years and Over by Age Groups Indicating Totals and Proportional Change from 1978-91 (thousands)

Age	1978	1981	1984	1988	1991
65-74					
Number	5017	5010	4653	4837	4792
%	100	99.8	92.7	96.4	95.5
75-84					
Number	2399	2568	2718	2795	2811
%	100	107.0	113.2	116.5	117.1
85+					
Number	529	559	600	659	736
%	100	105.7	113.4	124.6	139.1
65+					
Number	7945	8137	7971	8291	8339
%	100	102.4	100.3	104.3	105.0

Source: Office of Population Censuses and Surveys, *Population Projection 1978 to 2018* (United Kingdom), Table IVc, pp. 76-83.

Estimates for the year 1977-8 suggested that 33 per cent of people aged 65 years and over were living alone; for women aged 75 years and over, 50 per cent lived alone (Social Trends 1980: 90). This type of information, relating to changes in pattern of the population structure is important, not only from the aspect of disease that is likely to occur (chronic in the elderly), but for the planning of health services. Longevity means changes in life style and people who retire generally suffer a reduction in income and hence a change in life style. Loneliness can lead to depression, so that the epidemiologist considers not only the population structure but how it is made up and what effects changes in life style may have.

Changes in Life Style

Changes in life style since 1800 have been marked and working conditions, housing, nutrition and general affluence have helped to raise the standard of living for most people. Evidence shows, however, that for social classes IV and V improvement, as measured by mortality, has not increased proportionately to the improvement in the other social class groups. Poverty and poor housing do still exist and economic factors which have worldwide implications can change life styles adversely, as seen from the economic depression during the 1920s and more recently from the late 1970s.

The general trend has, however, been towards increased prosperity and with it greater mobility of manpower leading to a drift away from the country to industrialised towns. Even today many villages are socially isolated, consisting mainly in population terms of retired people. Property and trading brought new goods and technology, for example motor cars, alcohol and cigarettes and changes in habit and social acceptability created consumer markets for these products, which are now having serious implications in the population.

Thirty-two per cent of all motor vehicle drivers killed in road accidents in 1978 had blood alcohol levels over the legal limit and the cost of all road accidents in Great Britain in 1978 was £1,614 million (Department of Transport 1980: xi-xii). Alcohol and its dangers are widely recognised but its social acceptability may have played an important part in preventing a total ban on drinking and driving in this country.

Cigarette smoking, as mentioned earlier, became a socially accepted and widely practised habit first by men and then by women. The two world wars brought social changes such that cigarettes became cheap and readily available and the consequences of smoking only become apparent by careful epidemiological studies. The effect of cigarette smoking is demonstrated in Table 2.6 which shows how the standardised mortality rates for lung cancer, which for males has remained largely unchanged, has shown a continued rise for females. The results of such epidemiological studies have contributed to further changes in life style and fewer people are now smoking than previously. Today the epidemiologist is concerned with the effect that unemployment may have on health where generally adverse changes in life style have occurred. Will there be a tendency for increased psychiatric disorders, suicides or even premature deaths from other causes because of these social changes occurring in life style due to the present recession?

Changes in life style may not always give the hoped for benefits. Development of new towns immediately after the war to rehouse people, particularly those from London, produced unexpected results. Young families attracted by the prospects of new housing and jobs moved away from their previous close-knit environment and family support. This separation led to an increased consultation rate for psychiatric problems, particularly depression.

Table 2.6: England and Wales: Deaths and Standardised Mortality Rates for Cancer of the Lung and Bronchus in Males and Females for Selected Years 1968-78

Sex	1968	1970	1974	1978
Male				
Deaths (thousands)	23.9	24.9	26.4	26.7
SMR	100	102	106	103
Female				
Deaths (thousands)	3.9	5.4	6.5	7.6
SMR	100	107	130	146

Note: 1968 is the base year = 100.
Source: Office and Population Censuses and Surveys, *Mortality Statistics 1978* (England and Wales) Tables 6 and 8, pp. 10-58, 60-63.

Society's own affluence has also created a demand for independence, particularly in terms of transport. In 1932 there were 2.2 million motor vehicles licensed, by 1960 the figure was 8.9 million, and in 1978 no less than 17.3 million. Put another way, for every three people in Great Britain there is one motor vehicle. Such changes bring about their own problems; 50 per cent of deaths in males aged 15-19 years are due to motor vehicle accidents and in 1980 in Great Britain 3,280 people under 35 years of age died from this cause alone (Smith 1982: 17). Change in life style has also involved the work-place and new technology has altered working practices, but this has required new industries to be developed to meet the demand for new products and occupational change has brought about its own problems.

Occupational Diseases

The association of the work-place with illness and deaths has been recognised for many centuries. Specific legislation was introduced into some industries to try and reduce mortality and morbidity. For example, in the agricultural industry two specific pieces of legislation were introduced in the nineteenth century (as mechanisation took place) to try and reduce accidents. These were the 1878 Threshing Machine Act and the 1897 Chaff-Cutting Machine (Accident) Act. Today the Health and Safety at Work (etc) Act 1974 aims to provide guidelines for maintaining the health of employees, but responsibility lies with both employer and employee.

The association between coal mining and pneumoconiosis is an example of an occupational disease which has been reduced through careful studies, both by the Medical Research Council and the National Coal Board (Lock and Smith 1976: 142-6). Another example of association between occupation and diseases of the chest is that of workers in the asbestos industry. Work by Doll (1955: 81-6) and Whitwell, Scott and Grimshaw (1977: 377-86) has shown an association between asbestos fibres, cancer and other chest diseases.

Information about occupational mortality and morbidity can, however, be difficult to obtain. The Registrar General uses decennial information (every ten years) about occupational mortality and this has been in operation since 1851, with the exception of 1941. This data records the occupation at the time of the censuses. The problem arises, however, that people change occupation and may move from one occupation to another, perhaps because of ill-health. If they record their second job at the time of the census and then subsequently die in that job, that job will be recorded on the death certificate. The condition from which they died, however, might have been caused by exposure to a hazard in their first job. For example, bladder cancer is known to be associated with the chemicals benzodine and napthylamine, both used in the manufacture of analine dye stuffs. It was, however, some 30 years after the manufacturing process had been in operation that the association between this process and bladder cancer became recognised.

Thus, in occupational disease the problem arises not only of identifying the causal agents, perhaps because of a possible long latent period between exposure and disease presentation, but because the person concerned could have changed his/her occupation. This does not mean the search for the distribution and determinants of occupational disease stops, the process is simply more complex.

A knowledge of the hazards can reduce not only mortality but also morbidity. The commonest cause of morbidity in industry is due to accidents. Research into the cause of occupational accidents and the introduction of legislation, education and engineering for safety has been able to reduce some of the risks. Table 2.7 shows the gradual reduction in the accident rates for four industries between 1973 and 1979. Agriculture and coal mining show quite marked reductions, which reflect a multifactorial approach to the problem of accident prevention, including new technology. Basically, however, this area of occupational disease lies very much in our own hands, for if we do not take risks, but carry out duties as advised, then we can all play a major part in changing the pattern of disease.

Table 2.7: Great Britain: Non-fatal Reported Accidents in Selected Industries 1975-79 per 100,000 Employees at Risk

Industry	1975	1976	1977	1978	1979
Agriculture	1,800	1,800	1,600	1,500	1,400
Coal Mining	20,900	20,000	19,500	18,900	16,800
Manufacturing Industry	3,500	3,500	3,600	3,600	3,300
Construction Industry	3,500	3,500	3,300	3,400	3,100

Source: Health and Safety Commission, *Report 1979-80* (Great Britain), Table 3, p. 52.

Summary

Today changes in the pattern of disease are as important as 150 years ago, but the pattern of change can be more easily monitored through the data available to the epidemiologist and the means to manipulate it through the use of computers. The change in the pattern of disease may be the first indicator of a problem, as was the increase in congenital abnormalities resulting from the use of the drug thalidomide by pregnant women. Changes in mortality may be indicators of changes in morbidity but any change may have consequences for the provision of health care services. As already suggested, the increasing proportion of elderly in our society, particularly those aged 85 years and over, will bring an increased dependence on our health care services. Thus, the epidemiologist is involved in the planning of future health care service provision based on the monitoring of change.

3 INTRODUCTION TO THE LANGUAGE OF EPIDEMIOLOGY

What is Epidemiology?

Epidemiology can be defined as the study of disease in defined populations. The word epidemiology comes from Greek *epi* among, *demos* the people, *logos* science. It concerns the distribution of disease and the cause, or aetiology, of disease and is the scientific basis for much of community medicine. As an illustration of the concept of epidemiology let us consider what may be implied if a sister on a surgical ward comments that she thinks that now there is more wound infection, after a particular type of operation, than in the past. How would an epidemiologist react to a statement of this sort? Firstly, this statement is a subjective one and an epidemiologist would like details of the *number* of cases of wound infection rather than the general opinion that there was 'more of it around'. The number of cases would be a more objective statement but suppose that the sister then consulted ward records and found that, in the previous year, there had been 75 cases of wound infection, compared with 50 cases in a similar period ten years ago. This, she might contend, confirmed her suspicions.

The epidemiologist, however, would want more information (he usually does!). As well as the number of cases of wound infection, it would be desirable to know the number of patients having that particular type of operation (that is, in epidemiological terms, the population from which the cases come). This is often referred to as the population 'at risk'. Over the ten year period, this number might have changed. The operation may have become more, or less, frequent. For many conditions the length of stay in hospital has shown a steady decrease over the years and this fact alone might enable a larger number of operations to be done in one surgical ward in any one year. If the epidemiologist knew both the numbers of the particular operations that were done, and the numbers of those that developed wound infection, the *proportion* of patients developing wound infection could be calculated. For this purely hypothetical example, the number of patients having the particular operation is shown in Table 3.1. In this illustration, the *number* of infected wounds has increased by 50 per cent (from 50 to 75 a year) but the number of operations has also increased and, in fact, the wound infection *rate* has fallen slightly (from 1 in 7 to 1 in 8 of all cases).

Table 3.1: Hypothetical Example of Wound Infection after a Surgical Operation

	Number of operations	Number of infected wounds	Percentage of wounds with infection
Ten years ago	350	50	14.3
Previous year	600	75	12.5

In this example, was the ward sister 'right' in saying that there is more wound infection after the particular surgical procedure, than previously? It really depends on the context of her remarks and how these were interpreted. If patients (or the press!) concluded that patients now have a higher risk of developing wound infection after a particular operation, then the original statement is not only misleading but incorrect. If, however, the statement was made to justify more dressings for such patients on a particular ward it may be correct, as the number of infected cases from the particular operation in the ward in a year has increased. One of the advantages of using an epidemiological approach is that statements made, and figures provided, are the appropriate ones for the problem being considered. One of the skills in epidemiology, indeed in all research, is to ask the correct questions and to frame the questions in such a way that an answer can be found. Of course, in this example, there are many other aspects of the problem that should also be considered. These include, for example, the ages of the patients having the particular operation, the definition of exactly what is meant by wound infection and how this was assessed. Both these factors may have changed over the ten year period thus, perhaps, making direct comparisons difficult and possibly invalid.

The epidemiologist combines the information of health professionals (doctors, nurses, social workers) about groups of individual patients and the information of demographers about populations, especially the age and sex structure of the population. The epidemiologist, therefore, uses both the numerator (the number of cases) and the denominator (the population) and generally works in terms of rates. In the example given above, for the latest year, the numerator is 75 (the number of infected wounds) and the denominator is 600 (the number of patients having the particular operation — this is the population 'at risk' as it is only those having the operation that are at risk of developing the wound infection). It should be noted that the population being studied in this example is not the general population living in a particular area but a group of patients, identified as having a particular operation. Although in many studies the epidemiologist may indeed use the total population of a town, a county or a country, in other studies the population studied is defined, not by geographical boundaries, but by some other factor. A population, in the epidemiological sense, is a group of individuals that share some common characteristic. In the case of the hypothetical wound infection study, this common characteristic is that all the patients had a particular operation. It was necessary to know, for each year of the study, how many such patients had the operation and developed wound infection, and also how many had the same operation but did not develop wound infection.

One of the difficulties in epidemiology is to get the appropriate information on both the numerator and the denominator. For example a frequently encountered problem is that hospitals may have good information on the cases that are admitted to them, but it is often less easy to determine the population from which these patients come. Catchment areas for hospitals are, and must be, indefinite. Some patients may come from many miles away while other patients, living close to the hospital where the study is being conducted, may obtain treatment at another more distant hospital. Further, many patients may not have hospital treatment at all. Thus, although there is some information on both the patients (numerator) and the population (the denominator) it is not quite comparable information and it is this that could sometimes make the calculations of rates misleading.

For many diseases, only a proportion of all cases are known to doctors. Of course for the more serious diseases (such as cancer and heart disease) all patients may eventually be known to doctors but, at any one point in time, many will be undiagnosed. Some individuals with heart disease may in fact die suddenly from the disease, before it is diagnosed by a doctor, but they might have had evidence of heart disease for many years before death, and this would have been discovered if special tests had been used to seek out such disease. With many less serious diseases, surveys of the general population will frequently discover many more cases of disease than are known to general practitioners, and very many more cases than are included in hospital statistics. For example surveys of the general population for migraine have shown that only about half the individuals with migraine have ever consulted a doctor for it. This finding, that many more cases occur in the population than are known before a survey, is sometimes referred to as the 'iceberg phenomenon', with the medical and nursing professions seeing only the tip of the iceberg of all disease in the community.

Sources of Epidemiological Information

Information for epidemiological studies may either come from routine statistics or from special *ad hoc* studies. In some epidemiological studies it is possible to use the information that has already been collected for other reasons or is collected routinely. There is a wide variety of information that can be used both for the cases and for the population from which the cases come. Much of this information is collected, and published by the Office of Population Censuses and Surveys. For example, in studying the mortality from ischaemic heart disease, the number of deaths in men and women in various age groups is published for each year. The details of the population, and in particular the total number of men and women in these age groups, is available at the time of the national census (and less accurately for the years between). Examples of some of the information from routine statistics are given in Table 3.2.

Table 3.2: Some of the Examples of Information from Routine Statistics Available to the Epidemiologist

(1) *National Census.* In England and Wales a census has been completed every ten years since 1801 (except 1941).

(2) *Registration of Births and Deaths.* In England and Wales this has been available since 1838. Much of this data is published annually by the Registrar General.

(3) *Occupational Information.* The numbers, and sometimes ages, of individuals in various occupations may be available from the national census (above), from professional or industrial bodies and employers and from Trade Unions.

(4) *Hospital Statistics.* Hospital Activity Analysis (HAA) was initiated in 1965 and includes all discharges and deaths in hospital. The Hospital In-patient Inquiry (HIPI) was initiated in 1953 for every tenth discharge or death in hospital. There are separate reports for mental illness (in-patient statistics from the Mental Health Inquiry), and maternity.

(5) *Notifications of Infectious and other Disease.* Since the nineteenth century certain infectious diseases have been notifiable and data are published regularly by the Registrar General. Some industrial diseases are notifiable to the Chief Inspector of Factories.

(6) *Special Registers.* These are special registers, kept nationally, for certain conditions. A cancer register has been kept since 1945 and this has been national since 1962. A register of congenital malformations, since the thalidomide tragedy, begun in 1964. There is a national register of the disabled and blind.

(7) *Social Security Statistics.* Statistics are published about the amount and causes of sickness absence.

However, for some studies either the information required is not available from routine statistics, or the routine statistics are not quite appropriate for the purpose. It is then necessary to collect the required information specially for the study. In such cases, rather than examine all the individuals in a population, a statistically chosen sample (sometimes a random sample) is selected from the total population and only this sample is investigated in the study. Then the conclusions reached from this sample are, with any corrections necessary, related back to the whole population. The various sorts of epidemiological survey are discussed in detail in Chapter 4.

Prevalence and Incidence

The words *prevalence* and *incidence* are often confused or may be used indiscriminately in many publications. However, to the epidemiologist they are used to describe two quite distinct concepts. *Prevalence* is the proportion of existing cases of a disease in a population (Table 3.3). For example a survey of tuberculosis may show that in a population of 20,000 people there were four cases of tuberculosis, giving a prevalence of 1 in 5,000. This is an example of a *point prevalence*, because all four cases of tuberculosis were present at the time of the survey. However, for some conditions a point prevalence may not be an appropriate figure. For example, it would be difficult to measure the point prevalence of headache (that is the proportion of the population suffering from headache at one point in time) and, in any case, the figure would not be of much use. For headache, a *period prevalence* is the usual method of measurement and this will include all individuals who have had a headache at any time during a defined period of time. This period of time can be a week, a month or a year or is sometimes expressed as a life-time prevalence when anyone with the condition, at any time, is included. Prevalence is thus a *state* (the proportion of a population with a disease).

Table 3.3: The Difference Between Prevalence and Incidence

$$\text{Prevalence} = \frac{\text{Number of persons with a disease}}{\text{Total number in population}}$$

$$\text{Incidence} = \frac{\text{Number of persons developing a disease in a defined period of time}}{\text{Total number in population}}$$

Incidence is something quite different. It describes, not a state, but an *event* which is the rate of new cases developing in a population over a period of time (Table 3.3). In general it is more difficult to measure incidence than prevalence as it is necessary to know in a defined population the number *without the disease* at one point in time (the beginning), who *develop* the condition during a defined period of time. The relationship between point prevalence, period prevalence and incidence is shown in Figure 3.1. It is obvious that the relationship depends on the duration of the disease and the longer the duration, for any given incidence, the higher will be the point prevalence. This is sometimes expressed as:

Prevalence = Incidence x Duration

Figure 3.1: Relationship Between Prevalence and Incidence

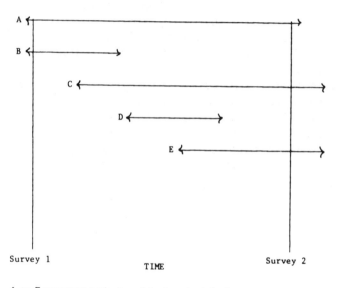

A to E represent patients and the length of the line represents the duration of the disease.

At Survey 1, there are two cases of the disease (A and B) for the point prevalence.

At Survey 2, there are three cases of the disease (A, C and D) for the point prevalence.

The incidence, between Surveys 1 and 2, includes cases C and E (and also D if the study can detect cases occurring between the two surveys who get better before the second survey).

The period prevalence, between Surveys 1 and 2, includes A, B, C, D and E as all these cases had, or developed, the disease during this period.

So far, we have expressed prevalence and incidence as rates and these may be expressed as per hundred, per thousand or in any other convenient way. Yet a comparison of rates, between two studies, may be misleading if the two survey populations were different, for example in their age distribution or sex ratio. It is for this reason that epidemiologists 'break down' their total populations and present their results in small age groups (perhaps five or ten year age groups). Also, as most diseases have different prevalences and incidences in males and females, the results are best presented separately for each sex. Table 3.4 gives a hypothetical example of a disease with the same overall prevalence in two age groups combined in men and in women (both 10 per cent). However, the prevalence in each age group separately shows that the prevalence is higher in men (5 per cent compared with 4 per cent at 25-34 years and 15 per cent compared with 11.2 per cent at 65-74 years). The reason for these findings is of course the fact that, in both sexes, the disease increases with age and that there are relatively more women in the older age group. It illustrates that crude rates (with all ages combined) may be misleading and show why age-specific (usually in age groups of five and ten years or similar) and sex-specific rates are preferable.

Table 3.4: Prevalence of Disease in Two Age Groups

	Age group (years)		Total
	25-34	65-74	
Number of men with disease	5	15	20
Population at risk	100	100	200
Number of women with disease	2	28	30
Population at risk	50	250	300

The overall prevalence rate is 10 per cent for both sexes but this hides the fact that it is lower in both age groups of women.

	Age group (years)		Total
	25-34	65-74	
Prevalence in men	5%	15%	10%
Prevalence in women	4%	11.2%	10%

Why Use Epidemiology? Epidemiology has several uses and it is the underlying discipline when considering the health and disease of populations. It developed in this country partly at least because routine information was available in some areas about births and deaths. Its first pioneer was not a medical man but a London haberdasher, John Graunt, who over three hundred years ago was the first person to notice that the number of births and deaths of males exceeded those of females, and who studied mortality from several diseases. During the nineteenth century epidemiology flourished with the increasing number of routine statistics that became available. Epidemiological studies concentrated on infectious disease which caused most of the deaths in childhood and younger adults. During the last 30 years epidemiology in this country has concentrated on non-infectious disease, as these conditions are now the main causes of morbidity and mortality.

The first use of epidemiology, therefore, was its use in determining the cause of disease. Even when the exact cause of the disease is not known, epidemiology can often identify certain groups of individuals who are at high risk of developing the disease. Epidemiology has shown that for several infectious diseases, mortality was falling before the organism responsible for the cause of the disease was identified. This was the case for tuberculosis and for cholera. Koch's discovery of the cause of tuberculosis, the tubercle bacillus, in 1882 was a historic event in the history of medicine. Yet this great discovery had little or no direct effect on mortality from tuberculosis, which was falling for many years before 1882 and continued to fall, at about the same rate, after 1882. Farr and Snow had clearly linked the mortality from cholera to contaminated drinking water (see Chapter 2) in the 1850s; action was taken and mortality from cholera fell. Yet the cause of cholera was not discovered until 1883 when Koch identified the cholera vibrio, a quarter of a century after Snow's death. We still do not know exactly what it is in cigarettes that causes chronic bronchitis and lung cancer but we do know if people give up smoking, or even cut down on the number smoked, morbidity and mortality are substantially reduced. Epidemiology is, therefore, important in determining the cause of disease and can be of great use even if the exact details of the pathogenesis are not understood.

Epidemiology has helped in evaluating treatments and in evaluating the organisation and running of health services. These aspects of epidemiology will be discussed later, as will the uses of epidemiology in planning health care.

4 TYPES OF STUDIES USED IN EPIDEMIOLOGICAL INVESTIGATIONS

Introduction

All epidemiological studies are, by definition, carried out in defined, or at least definable, populations. There have been several attempts to classify epidemiological studies into different types and this has its practical uses, as if the type of study is known, one has some idea about the advantages, and limitations, of the method used. No classification of surveys is completely satisfactory. Each study is best thought through and designed on its merits depending on the particular situation rather than being made to fit in to one or other of the types of surveys of any classification. One obvious division of surveys is to separate those where individuals are seen only once and those where individuals are followed up over time. This can be done for both *descriptive surveys* and for *analytical surveys* where a particular idea or hypothesis is being investigated (Table 4.1). The third type of epidemiological survey is the *experimental study* where the division of individuals into two or more groups may be done by randomisation.

Table 4.1: Types of Epidemiological Survey

	Observations made at one point in time	Observations made at more than one point in time
Descriptive surveys	Cross-sectional survey	Longitudinal survey
Analytical surveys	Case-control study	Cohort study
Experimental study	—	Experimental study

Descriptive Surveys

Descriptive surveys are, as their name implies, descriptions of the amount and distribution of diseases in populations. The survey can include the whole population, or more usually a sample of the population is selected for special study (see Chapter 5). Such studies describe three main characteristics: *who* is affected, *where* the disease occurs and *when* the disease occurs.

When investigating *who* gets a disease, the epidemiologist is particularly concerned with the age and sex of the sufferers, as most diseases vary greatly in different age groups and in men and women. As many diseases occur more frequently in certain social classes or socio-economic groups, information on this is also frequently obtained in the survey. Other aspects that may be important in describing who gets diseases include marital state and sometimes family size, birth order and other demographic factors.

Descriptive surveys measure *where* diseases occur. Diseases do not have a fixed incidence and prevalence, but vary. The places of frequent occurrence may be related to natural boundaries, such as mountain ranges, rivers or islands or they may have man-made or political boundaries. Some infectious diseases occur almost entirely in the tropics and frequently in only certain parts of the tropics. The study of geographical pathology may give a clue to the cause of some diseases and the distribution of the disease must be related to the distribution of its possible cause. For example, endemic goitre has been found to be associated with inland areas deficient in iodine. Other diseases may have a striking, if complex, geographical distribution. Multiple sclerosis, a remitting but usually progressive neurological disorder of young adults, is rare in the tropics but increases with distance from the tropics in both northern and southern hemispheres. More locally, diseases may vary between nearby urban and rural areas and, within an urban area, may be concentrated in the locality of, for example, a factory producing pollution.

The third main characteristic described in such surveys is *when* the disease occurs. Most diseases, both infectious and non-infectious, show slow variations in incidence over long periods of time; these long-term changes are known as secular trends. For example, in Britain tuberculosis has been declining in incidence for about a hundred and fifty years whereas coronary heart disease has increased greatly during the twentieth century. Some diseases show variations in frequency at regular (usually shorter) intervals; an example of these changes are those diseases that have an annual or seasonal pattern, e.g. hay fever, or occur with high frequency at fairly regular intervals every two or three years, e.g. measles. These short-term patterns are known as cyclic changes.

The methods used in descriptive surveys depend on the disease being studied. The surveys may involve only a questionnaire or basic measurements such as height, weight, blood pressure, or they may include blood tests, lung function tests and other more detailed investigations. As a rule, tests used in epidemiology are fairly simple as they normally have to be fairly cheap and capable of being applied to large samples of the population. As a high response rate is desirable, the tests used must also be acceptable to the general population. They must also be reasonably cheap and accurate (Table 4.2).

Table 4.2: Desirable Characteristics of Tests used in Epidemiological Surveys

Characteristic	Reason
Acceptable	As high response rate is desirable
Low cost	As large numbers are usually done
Accurate	As inaccuracies may increase cost, anxiety and make study less valid.

Descriptive studies sometimes do not measure diseases, but some aspect related to disease. Figure 4.1 shows the proportion of women who have had dysuria (defined as pain or burning on urination) in the previous year (a *period* prevalence). This is one of the symptoms of infection of the urinary tract but from the study it was not possible to be certain, in each instance, whether there was indeed other evidence of urinary tract infection. The figure shows, rather unexpectedly, that this symptom was not related to age (at least within the range studied), it also shows that, when only those women who consulted a doctor are considered, the symptom appears more frequent in younger women, which is the textbook picture of urinary tract infection. Figure 4.1 therefore shows one of the reasons for conducting epidemiological studies in the general population rather than relying on information available to health professionals. With regard to dysuria, information from general practitioners' surgeries would have considerably underestimated the prevalence. More than this, the information from general practitioners would have suggested that the prevalence of dysuria varied with age, whereas the epidemiological survey suggested that this was not so. One must always keep in mind that routinely available statistics may not only be inaccurate estimates of the frequency of disease but that their data may be *biased*. In the case of the information shown in Figure 4.1, the data which would have been available from doctors would have given a misleading idea of the effect of age on the prevalence of dysuria.

Descriptive surveys are known as cross-sectional when they are done at one point in time. If, however, they are repeated on the same population sample they are known as longitudinal studies. As people change addresses, longitudinal studies are more difficult to do, but such studies add extra dimensions to the information that can be obtained. They can be used to see what happens to people with particular diseases or particular symptoms.

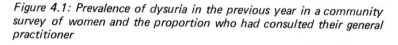

Figure 4.1: Prevalence of dysuria in the previous year in a community survey of women and the proportion who had consulted their general practitioner

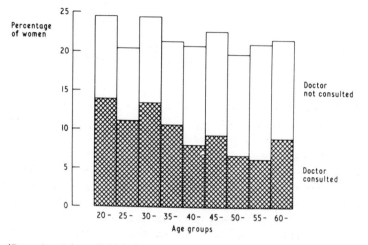

(Reproduced from *British Journal of Preventive and Social Medicine*, 1969, 23, 263).

Analytical Studies

Analytical studies test a particular hypothesis (or idea) about the cause of disease. They are of two types, depending on whether or not the subjects are seen at more than one point in time (Table 4.1). The simplest analytical study is known as the case-control study. In these studies patients with a particular disease (cases) are compared with controls who do not have the disease; differences in the previous experience of the cases and controls are sought. For example, in an early study by Doll and Hill (1950: 739-48) to examine whether smoking cigarettes was associated with lung cancer, patients with lung cancer, and patients with other diagnoses, were questioned about their previous smoking habits. The study showed a deficiency of non-smokers and an excess of heavy smokers in the lung cancer group. Case-control studies are generally relatively quick and cheap to do but may suffer from selection of inappropriate controls. It is usual for the controls to be *matched* with the cases. This is done for example by selecting controls of the same age and sex as the patients. Such selection is often difficult and controversial (MacMahon and Pugh 1970).

The other type of analytic study is the cohort study, where a group or groups of individuals are followed up over a period of time to see whether or not they develop particular diseases. In the case of the cigarette hypothesis for lung cancer, Doll and Hill obtained the smoking habits of doctors by obtaining their names from the medical register and writing to them with a questionnaire. These doctors were then followed up and, as they died, copies of the death certificates were obtained. This study revealed that cigarette smokers identified in the initial survey had a higher death rate than did non-smokers. Further, among the smokers, the death rates were higher among the heavy smokers than among those who had smoked less (Doll and Hill 1964).

The word *cohort* comes from the Latin meaning a large group of warriors or persons banded together. A cohort is thus a group of people with some common characteristic, such as year of birth, and a cohort study is the study of such a population over a period of time. Cohort studies are generally scientifically more valid than case-control studies, but they often take much longer to do and are, therefore, more expensive. They are generally inappropriate for rare diseases as the number of individuals to be studied would have to be very large in order to obtain enough cases developing the disease in a reasonable period of time.

Both types of analytical study look at the association between a disease and the possible cause. Let us assume that the disease has a single cause (this is in fact unusual as the cause of disease is really multifactorial). Table 4.3 shows that where populations are exposed to the possible cause the disease develops, but where they are not exposed the disease is absent. In the case-control study one starts with two groups; one with the disease (the cases) and one without (the controls). By questions, or other methods, one looks *backwards* to see what proportion in each of the two groups were exposed to the possible cause in the past. In cohort studies, however, one starts with one or more populations, some individuals from which will be exposed to the possible cause, and measures over time the proportion who develop the disease.

Table 4.3: Details of Analytical Studies (see text)

		Case-control study	
		Disease present	
Cohort Study		Yes	No
	Exposure to	+	−
	possible cause	−	+

Some classifications of surveys use the terms *prospective* and *retrospective* but these terms can, and do, cause confusion and are therefore usually better avoided. It is true that case-control studies are always retrospective. Cohort studies, however, can be either prospective or retrospective. An example of a retrospective cohort study might, for instance, be an investigation into the risk of asbestos in a population working in a factory. A factory might have names and details of all the employees on its pay roll in 1950. The cohort is, therefore, this population of employees who could then be followed up, perhaps to 1980, and the number developing various forms of cancer identified. Due to the good records of the company it is, therefore, possible to do an 'instantaneous' thirty year follow-up. (Incidentally, this illustrates the epidemiological maxim 'where money changes hands, good records are kept'). This survey has all the advantages of a cohort study and is sometimes known as the historical cohort or, confusingly, a prospective survey carried out in a retrospective manner.

Experimental Studies

Experimental studies are usually concerned with the treatment of disease, but may also be used to assess the prevention of disease and also its cause. In their most developed form experimental studies use random allocation into two or more groups. These are variously known as clinical trials or randomised trials (and sometimes as controlled trials). Obviously such trials, carried out in the general population (or anywhere else), raise important, and sometimes difficult, ethical issues. Nevertheless randomised trials are accepted as powerful techniques which can be used, for example, to compare two or more treatments where differences are not apparent as a result of other methods of assessment. It is important to realise that it is where other methods of assessment are unsatisfactory, or incomplete, that randomised trials are indicated. A criticism sometimes made of randomised trials is that they have never discovered a *really* important advance in medicine. Much depends on what is considered really important, but because of the way that they are used a striking advance would not be expected. If a new treatment was found always to be successful in a disease that was previously invariably fatal, it would not be necessary to do a randomised trial!

A randomised trial is a technique to experimentally test a hypothesis using random allocation and invariably involves intervention by the researchers. The division into two or more groups is done by some method independent of human choice (by using tables of random numbers).

Although the use of strict randomisation is virtually confined to the second half of the twentieth century, the ideas behind these studies are much older. Indeed it has been pointed out that any treatment for any individual patient is really a 'trial', as one is not certain of the results that will be obtained because each patient is different. In 1753 Lind reported treating twelve patients with scurvy at sea ('their cases were as similar as I could have them'), by six different methods. Those treated with oranges and lemons made a dramatic recovery and one was 'appointed nurse to the rest of the sick'. Although the allocation of these six treatments does not appear to have been randomised, in essence the study was a very early example of a clinical trial.

Randomisation produces two or more groups that are more or less similar for all the characteristics thought to be important in the study. For example, age may be related to outcome of treatment and two randomised groups will have similar age structures (subject only to chance fluctuations which become less important with larger numbers). Of possibly greater importance is the fact that the two groups produced by randomisation should be similar for other characteristics, including any characteristics that are not even known to medical science at the time of the study. Obviously it is not possible to match, or allow for, such characteristics, yet these may well be important. It is these characteristics of randomised trials that make them such a scientifically valid and powerful tool. However, the limitations of randomised trials should also be kept in mind. Just because a particular result is obtained from a randomised trial it does not mean that the result is appropriate in all circumstances. Randomised trials set out to answer one (or sometimes a few) questions and, therefore, give answers that are specific. For example, if a randomised trial did not show an advantage of a particular new drug over a placebo (or inert substance), the conclusion should be that in that dose, given by that route (e.g. orally), at that frequency (say, three times a day), for that duration (say, five days), in that group of patients and using the outcome measured, the efficacy of the new drug was not established. We do not know if the result would have been different if the dose was changed, if the route of administration was different, if the frequency of administration was altered, if the duration was longer or if a different population of patients was investigated.

The outcome measured is also important and assessment may be different if symptoms or bacteriological cure, for example, are measured. The outcome may also depend on when the measurement is made (short term or long term). These questions cannot all be answered at once and therefore very large numbers of randomised trials may be necessary, even investigating a single drug. This does not mean that randomised trials are not useful but illustrates that, by their nature, they give specific answers to specific questions. As a method of investigation for these specific questions randomised studies are unrivalled.

The word randomised refers, of course, to just one aspect of the study, the method of allocation into the groups. Even a randomised study can give a misleading result if other aspects of the study are not designed and completed properly. A few of these are considered below, and are important in many epidemiological and clinical studies and not just in randomised trials.

Two other types of study, although not randomised, may come under the general description of experimental studies. The first is the *uncontrolled experiment*. Here there is an intervention 'as an experiment', but there is either no control or an inadequate control. Sometimes such studies are 'before and after' studies where changes are assessed before and after the introduction of a new treatment or new management. Scientifically such studies are variable but must always be interpreted with extreme care, as other things too may have changed.

Finally, there are the *natural experiments*. The classic example is Dr John Snow's observations on cholera in the mid-nineteenth century in London. Snow noted that cholera rates were higher amongst those obtaining their drinking water from one water company compared with those supplied by its rival (Table 4.4). Yet the two groups were otherwise similar; 'a few houses are supplied by one Company and a few by the other, according to the decision of the owner or occupier at that time when the Water Companies were in active competition'. From his careful observations, Snow deduced that the population who obtained their water from lower down the River Thames, who were supplied with 'water containing the sewage of London and, amongst it, whatever might have come from the cholera patients', experienced the higher death rate from cholera. Snow did not know about the cholera vibrio (which was not identified by Koch until 1883), but discovered enough about cholera to prevent the disease. Snow's study was not randomised but, as he said, 'it is obvious that no experiment could have been devised which would more thoroughly test the effect of water supply on the progress of cholera than this, which circumstances placed ready-made before the observer'. It was Snow's appreciation that this natural experiment was taking place that contributed to his lasting fame. The advantages of natural experiments are that they may be much less costly than randomised ones, they may avoid ethical problems, and they may already have taken place, so that the results are not

subjected to the biased recording which may occur with planned inter-
ventions.

*Table 4.4: Mortality from Cholera 8 July to 26 August 1854 in Districts
Served by Two Water Companies*

Water Company	Population 1851 Census	Number of Deaths	Death rate per 1000 Population
Southwark and Vauxhall	98,862	419	4.24
Lambeth	154,615	80	0.52

Some Important Aspects of Epidemiological Studies

The *selection* of subjects into any study is important. A study which is
done on hospital patients may give different results from one conducted
in a health centre, which in turn may give different results from one
conducted in the general population. All may be correct for the population studied and each may be appropriate for different circumstances,
however, it may be wrong to extrapolate from one population group to
another. For example, most headaches in the general population are
relieved by taking aspirin but a study of the efficacy of aspirin in neurological out-patients presenting with headache is likely to show that
aspirin is much less useful. This is because individuals with headaches
that are cured by aspirin are less likely to go to their general practitioner and also less likely to be referred on to a neurological specialist.
Patients who are referred to a neurologist are, therefore, highly *selected*,
are not typical of all headache sufferers, are less likely to respond to
aspirin and are more likely to have headaches caused by serious underlying conditions. The efficacy of aspirin in one population cannot be
extrapolated to another different population.

In any study the *response rate* and *drop-out rate* (the proportion of
those that enter a study but do not remain in it) are important. Ideally
the response rate should be high and the drop-out rate should be low.
These features are desirable, not just because the total numbers available for study are increased, but because those who refuse, or drop out,
may be different from those who co-operate, and the remaining sample
may become biased (not typical of the original population).

If possible, the criteria used in epidemiological studies should be
objective rather than *subjective*. For example, with hypertension, the
blood pressure should be measured and individuals should not just be

categorised as normal and hypertensive. Even the measurement of blood pressure with a mercurial sphygmomanometer is only an estimation of the actual pressure within the artery. It will be assessed differently by different observers (*inter-observer variation*) and even by the same observer on different occasions (*intra-observer variation*). These variations are distinct from the variations in pressure that occur over time, within the same individual, and are simply due to the observer making slightly different estimates of the value when the sounds appear or disappear. Usually this intra-observer variation will show roughly equal numbers above and below a mean value, which will be that observer's best estimate of the pressure. In clinical practice, the inter-observer variation in blood pressure is usually of little or no consequence. If one observer makes a blood pressure 180/125 mm Hg and another makes it 170/120, the patient is obviously hypertensive. In epidemiological studies, however, even a very small inter-observer variation, if it is consistent, may create great problems. This is because inter-observer variation is not random but systematic, with one observer repeatedly obtaining slightly higher results than the other. If blood pressures are measured among the employees of two factories, each by its own occupational nurse, a small but consistent difference in the means may be found. If this is a true difference between the blood pressures of the employees, it may be important from the point of view of the cause of hypertension. It may, however, simply reflect the inter-observer difference between the blood pressure readings of the two nurses. This possibility should have been taken into account when the study was designed, either by testing for inter-observer differences before the survey or by using a single observer. Observer variation is also known as *observer error* because, if the results are different, at least one of them must be wrong!

If the measurement is subjective, but also even if it is fairly objective, it is desirable to make the observations *blindly*, that is with the observer not knowing the group which each subject is from when making the observations. This may be important as it can eliminate bias from the results. Where the subject too does not know if the drug taken was the active one, or the placebo, the study is described as *double-blind*. This is a desirable feature, especially with subjective assessments, as both subjects and observers are often influenced by the results that they are expecting.

5 DRAWING A SAMPLE FOR A STUDY

The Need for a Sample

In Chapter 1 reference was made to the introduction in 1800 of the Population Act which enabled central government, through the Registrar General, to carry out a census of the total population of England and Wales every ten years. The last census was in 1981, cost over £10 million and the results of the analysis of the data are only just becoming available — some take as many as three years to appear. Clearly, this type of study of a whole population is expensive both in actual financial costs as well as manpower, and has to be able to handle large amounts of data (information) which today are analysed by computers. For most people who wish to study a particular problem in a population, resources are not usually available to undertake the study on the whole population and, therefore, they carry out a study on a 'sample' of the population.

Sampling implies using only a proportion of the whole population and as such introduces a factor termed 'sampling error'. This error arises simply because the investigator is not using the whole population and no matter how complete the sample is the error remains. (The investigator can allow statistically for the sampling error and can set limits for the error and try and compensate for them, as will be outlined later.) A sample, therefore, is simply any part of a defined population.

Sampling is used not only because of the resource implications but also because, in trying to study whole populations, inevitably there will be a loss of information for a number of reasons. These may include the fact that people are away at the time of the census, are ill, or just refuse to participate. In effect, therefore, the investigator is left in any case with a sample of the whole population, but doesn't know how representative it is of the whole. On the other hand, the properly drawn sample, even with its inherent sampling error, for which some allowance can be made, because it is smaller in size, may allow a more complete collection of information which may be more valuable than a more incomplete study of the whole population. As indicated previously, however, a sample does have inherent in it the error termed the sampling error, and the investigator tries to reduce or set limits for this error to allow inferences to be made about the whole population, based on the results collected in the sample.

The Sample

Before an investigator proceeds with a study a number of questions need to be considered. These include the type of information that is required, whether sampling is a suitable method for investigating the problem and, if sampling is an acceptable method, what sample size is required to be representative of the whole population. The type of sampling method to be adopted will then be an important consideration. Before considering the methods, some basic aspects of the sample itself need to be considered.

Reduction of Bias

One of the fundamental principles of drawing a random sample from a whole population is that every person or characteristic in that population has an equal chance of appearing in the sample. Bias is the concept that, intentionally or unintentionally, the equal chance to appear has *not* occurred. For an example, an investigator wishes to interview a sample of student nurses (studying for their state registration examination) concerning their smoking habits. To obtain the sample the investigator meets a class of students and chooses 30 from the class. Is this a representative sample of the student nurses at that hospital?

This sample could have a number of intentional or unintentional biases relating to the population of nurses in it. The class would probably be limited to a particular year of entry and hence stage in training and, therefore, is not representative of all student nurses. The investigator might have been influenced by the colour of hair of the students, choosing those with dark rather than light colour. In the first case the bias is unintentional, but obviously the group is not representative of the whole population of student nurses and, therefore, not everybody had an equal opportunity to appear in the sample. In the second case the bias could be intentional, the investigator preferring dark to light hair-coloured ones, and it could be that these people smoked more often than light haired nurses. Further, the nurses who smoke heavily are more likely to be ill with respiratory disease and hence will not be interviewed. Whilst these are extreme examples they illustrate the problem that bias can cause, whether intentional or unintentional. To avoid bias, sampling methods have been devised to overcome this problem and are governed by agreed sets of principles in drawing the sample.

Defining the Population

An important feature of any study is to define the whole population
in which the study is to be carried out and from which the sample is
to be drawn. For example, if an investigator wished to study smoking
habits amongst nurses, because of the different sub-groups of nurses
within the total profession, there would need to be a definition of
which group of nurses was to form the population to be studied. This
could be all whole- or part-time nurses employed in a particular district
health authority, irrespective of grade. This would, therefore, include
auxiliary, hospital, community and administrative nursing staff. Alter-
natively, the study could be confined to all whole- or part-time nurses
employed in a regional health authority as midwives (excluding pupil
midwives) who hold the State Certificate of Midwifery. In the two
examples the whole population to be studied is defined and a sample
can be drawn from that defined population. Any inference from the
sample would relate only to the defined whole population from which
the sample was drawn. The population need not, however, be people,
and may be comprised of birth weights, blood pressures or other parameters.

Size of Sample

The size of the sample required basically depends on the prevalence, or
amount, of the characteristic or disease in the whole population. In
some studies, however, the prevalence of the characteristic or disease
under investigation may not be known, in which case a judgement has
to be made as to the sample size, and this may depend on the amount
of resource available for the study. Where the prevalence is known
then it is possible, by using a mathematical equation, to calculate the
size of the sample and at the same time to set limits as to the required
accuracy that the sample will reflect of the whole population. In
practice, the investigator would discuss the aspects of sample size with
a statistician, who would also be asked for advice during all stages of
the study and this practice is recommended to readers to ensure that
the sample is as representative as possible of the defined whole population. Often it is possible to find from the literature other studies of
the characteristic or disease and to obtain some estimate from those
of the prevalence of the condition. For example, in respect of the
presence of cigarette smoking amongst nurses, the following results
have been obtained from various studies: 37.3 per cent of nurses in a

study of registered nurses in America (Green 1970: 1936-8), 39 per cent amongst student nurses in Australia (Niel, Clark and Muller 1980: 47-8) and 24-45 per cent amongst nurses in Scotland (Small and Tucker 1978: 1878-9). In deciding on the sample size the results quoted above would have to be taken in the context of the whole population to which the sample results referred.

When estimating the sample size required to determine the prevalence of a particular condition, a major determinant is the precision specified for the estimate. The sample size is inversely proportional to the square of a measure of the precision. For example, if we required to know the prevalence to be within 10 per cent of our estimate, then the sample size is proportional to $1/0.1^2 = 100$. If instead we specified 5 per cent, e.g. an estimate of 25 per cent, and the true value to be between 20-30 per cent, then the sample size is proportional to $1/0.05^2 = 400$. Thus to double the precision we have to quadruple the sample size.

Enumerating the Whole Population

Before the investigator in any study draws a sample, the whole population (previously defined) requires to be listed and enumerated; a complete list of such nurses is known as the sampling frame. For example, in the study of smoking habits amongst nurses in a district health authority, each individual nurse would be allocated a number. This procedure is essential to ensure that when the whole population is sampled each person has an equal chance of appearing in the sample, based on the sampling methods.

Methods of Sampling

There are a number of methods of sampling available to the investigator and the method chosen depends to some extent on the size of the whole population to be studied. In each step of the different methods the whole population needs to be enumerated. The different methods of sampling will be discussed individually.

Simple Random Sampling

This method is generally applicable to small whole populations of less than one thousand, where enumeration is not difficult and the sample can be drawn using random number tables. Random number tables are, as they imply, sets of tables of numbers produced randomly, for example by a computer. Table 5.2 illustrates part of a page of a random number table. To draw a sample of the size required, the investigator may start anywhere in the table and move either across or down the table, provided that the movement is consistent. Each number obtained from the table will then be matched with the same number in the whole population and that person or characteristic will then form part of the sample population. The procedure continues until the appropriate sample size is drawn. Where by chance a number occurs twice during the course of using the tables then, in population studies of people, the number is discarded the second time and the next number taken. In studies of measurement, however, for example birth weights, then the convention is that the weight may be entered into the study again. In view of the different conventions the reader is recommended to consult with a statistician about the use of the random number table to ensure that the sample size is obtained correctly.

Table 5.2: Example of Random Numbers

03	47	43	73	86	39	96	47	36	61
97	74	24	67	72	32	81	14	57	20
16	76	62	27	66	96	96	68	27	31
55	95	36	35	64	31	62	43	09	90

Multi-stage Sampling

As the title suggests, in this method the whole population is sampled in stages, each stage being sampled randomly. This type of method is useful where large numbers are involved in the whole population. For example, if an investigator wished to study the prevalence of colour-blindness in boys aged 11-16 years, in State schools, in a particular county, then initially all State schools where boys of this age were educated could be enumerated. A random sample of these schools could then be drawn and this would form a sample of the total schools. From each of the sample schools, boys aged 11-16 would then be enumerated and equal sample sizes would then be drawn from each of the schools within the age group 11-16 years, on a random basis. In each procedure, therefore, enumeration took place and a random sample was drawn; every school and within each school every pupil had an equal chance of selection.

Stratified Sampling

This method is an extension of multi-stage sampling and is particularly useful when the disease or characteristic under observation is known to vary, for example, with age and sex. If an investigator wished to study the seat-belt wearing habit amongst National Health Service employees in a large district health authority and compare this habit with the general population, a simple random sample would produce a large number of females in the Health Service employees sample, since nearly 80 per cent of employees are females.

To overcome this difficulty, the nominal role of the district health authority could be divided into males and females, which gives two groups. It is known, however, that seat-belt wearing varies with age, older people being more likely to wear seat-belts than younger people, so that it would be necessary to stratify the two groups, males and females, by age using decennial (ten year) age groups. This stratification is illustrated in Figure 5.1. From each of the age group strata equal-sized random samples would then be drawn after enumerating the population in each of the age groups, both males and females. This again fulfils the principle of random sampling, namely that each individual has an equal chance of being in the sample within the age-sex group. Whilst this appears a complex method, it gives a more even distribution to the whole population under investigation and, in this case, females would not dominate the sample, and that individual age groups would have an equal chance of being represented in the sample.

Figure 5.1: Example of Stratified Sampling

Defined Population

(Personnel employed by a
District Health Authority)

First Strata

Males   Females

Second Strata

Age Groups

| 16-24 | 35-44 | 55-64 |
| 25-34 | 45-54 |

Systematic Sampling

This method of sampling is sometimes used when, for reasons beyond the control of the investigator, the whole population cannot be enumerated without a great deal of effort and resources which might preclude the study being undertaken at all. This method is sometimes employed when a small sample is required from a very large one, for example the electoral roll of a local authority district from which only a small sample is required. In this type of sampling, the investigator takes every nth name for the sample. For example, from an electoral roll of 60,000 a one in a hundred sample is required. This would require 600 people, but because of the way the electoral rolls are held it is easier to take every one hundredth name. To ensure an equal chance of every person being involved in the study the starting point is obtained randomly. For example, the seventeenth name may be obtained from the random number tables and subsequently the systematic sample would include the 117, 217, 317 until 600 names had been obtained.

This method does have limitations and can, in certain circumstances, produce bias. Thus, before using systematic sampling as a method, the investigator needs to consult with a statistician as to whether this is the most satisfactory method or whether some other method should be employed.

Quota Sampling

Quota sampling is a method of stratified sampling in which the selection within each strata is non-random, and it is this non-random element that constitutes its greatest weakness (Moser and Kalton 1972: 127). Quota sampling is a method often used by market research or opinion poll organisations and, using this method, interviewers who are employed to carry out the sampling are given instructions about certain characteristics, for example age, sex and social status, of the individuals to be selected. The proportions of the characteristics in the various subgroups are chosen to represent as far as possible the corresponding proportions in the whole population being studied. Thus, before quota sampling is used as a method, readers are recommended to consult with a statistician.

Sampling is a complex problem and care in deciding on the appropriate method is essential. Consultation with a statistician should be part of the process of establishing a study within a whole defined population and to discuss which method of sampling would be the most appropriate for the study concerned.

Problems in Sampling

A number of problems occur in the process of sampling. The investigator needs to realise the extent to which these problems can influence the results and hence the inferences that can be drawn from the sample to the whole population. These will be discussed individually.

Non-responders

In sampling a whole defined population, some of the people or measurements may not respond or not be available. In respect of studies of illness or habits amongst the population, non-response may occur for a variety of reasons. The person may be ill at the time of the study, on holiday or refuse to participate. The loss of these people or measurements does, however, reduce the randomness of the sample.

The tracing of the non-responders and the gathering of data from them is important and should be pursued wherever possible. In a survey on smoking, the non-responders may in fact be people who smoke and if they are lost from the sample the results would be biased. Non-response may also be due to poor design of the study, particularly if questionnaires are used. Inevitably, however, there will always be a number of non-responders and the investigator will need to decide whether their absence is likely to distort the sample in relation to the problem under study. The problem can be overcome by drawing a further small sub-sample from the non-responders and, by concentrating effort, attempting to achieve as near 100 per cent response as possible. Using this sub-sample data it would then be possible to compare these results with those from the original sample and examine the extent of the differences, if any.

Volunteers

Using volunteers to form a sample should, wherever possible, be avoided. Such groups may be atypical of the population as a whole and introduce bias. There are occasions, however, when the principle of true randomness has to be set aside in the interests of speed in obtaining a result. An example quoted by Barker and Rose (1979: 40) refers to the problem that a clinical pathologist may have in establishing the normal range of serum calcium as measured by a new method. In practice it is easier to use laboratory staff to obtain blood samples than to try and obtain random samples of blood from a defined population. Even if such a population could be found, again it would be easier to call for volunteers than to draw a random sample because of the problem of non-responders. Whilst accepting that these are short cuts, and that there are potential dangers in using volunteers, it may be appropriate for the occasion. The use of volunteers does, therefore, present risks and has been shown to produce biased results, but provided that this is accepted and understood and the shortcomings realised, expediency may dictate its use. Where possible the results obtained by this short-cut method should be compared with those obtained from a more randomly-based sample.

Confidence in the Sample's Results

From the sample, the investigator wishes to draw inferences about the whole population. In the section on sample size the question of setting the limits which were acceptable was outlined briefly, but this made the assumption that information about the possible prevalence or proportion of the disease or characteristic in the population was known. In some studies the investigator is actually trying to determine the extent of the disease or characteristic with no previous knowledge.

In this instance the results from his sample may give some indication of whether the inference that can be drawn about the whole population is acceptable. Bradford-Hill (1966: 22) gives the example that deafness was found in 18 per cent of a sample of a population. This value, when applied to the whole population, suggests that the proportion of people with deafness lies between the interval of 10 to 26 per cent, the sample value of 18 being the average of these values. If this interval is too large then a larger sample of the whole population should be drawn. Thus, in looking at the confidence with which the sample results can be used to draw inferences about the general population, the sample size becomes a critical factor. Readers are therefore advised to consult a statistician about the question of the sample size.

In summary, a sample can be used to study a whole defined population even though the sample itself introduces the sampling error (which can be estimated) provided that basic rules are followed. The sample, because of its small size, can become very precise if attention is paid to reducing the proportion of non-responders (absence of information). The basis of drawing a sample is one of randomness, allowing every person or measurement in the whole defined population to have an equal chance or known chance of appearing in the sample. For this purpose, random number tables provide the means of effecting the opportunity for everybody to have an equal chance of appearing in the sample. Before starting to draw a sample we would suggest that the aid of a statistician is sought to ensure that the study design is satisfactory, that the method of sampling which is being proposed will satisfy the necessary criteria and the sample will be appropriate for the population under study.

6 SIMPLE STATISTICS USED IN COMMUNITY MEDICINE

Certain basic statistical concepts are important in any understanding of the data that must be examined in community medicine. Some people may still shudder at the mention of the word *statistics*. While those researchers contributing to new knowledge by the presentation of papers and reports must have a considerable knowledge of statistics and access to a statistician, everyone reading the health literature should be able to appreciate certain statistical concepts. If they cannot do so, they really cannot assess the relevance and importance of many pieces of research. It is not the intention of this chapter to compete with the many statistical textbooks that can be used by health professionals. Its purpose is to try and present briefly some statistical concepts in the hope that the reader will find these useful in reading the statistical sections of reports. Much of this statistical material can in fact be understood, sometimes perhaps only partially understood, with a surprisingly scanty knowledge of statistics and even this scanty knowledge should be enough to enable the reader to understand the authors' conclusions.

Probability

'Significantly more women than men suffer from urinary tract infections ($p < 0.05$, two-tailed test).'

If a survey made the above conclusion the reader could either accept the conclusion that more women than men suffer from urinary tract infections and ignore the statistical jargon contained in the brackets, or could try and understand what the jargon means. It does in fact describe how confident the authors are about the truth of their findings. The reasoning behind this statement is as follows. In this hypothetical survey, the authors have assumed that there is no difference in the prevalence of such infections in men and women and completed a survey on, say, 1000 individuals. The prevalence of such infections found in the survey in men and women is likely to differ, if only on the grounds of chance. The figure $p < 0.05$ indicates that a difference at least as great as that observed would occur less than five times in a hundred. That is the odds are 19 to 1 against this finding if there were no differences in the number of urinary tract infections in men and women. The other again arbitrary statistical level used frequently in medicine is $p < 0.01$. Here the odds of this outcome are less than 99 to 1, again assuming no real difference. Instead of quoting the arbitrary levels $p < 0.05$ and $p < 0.01$, sometimes authors quote the actual significance levels, e.g. $p = 0.032$, where the level of significance lies between $p < 0.05$ and $p < 0.01$.

Rather than accept that an unlikely event has occurred, the authors reach the more likely conclusion that urinary tract infections are more frequent in women. However, if the evidence for this statement is based only on this one study, which was based only on a sample of 1000, it just might be wrong (due to chance). What the jargon tells us is that it is statistically unlikely to be wrong (less than 1 in 20 or 1 in 100 in the cases given). Although the possible p values are a continuum, arbitrary levels are considered statistically significant (often $p < 0.05$ or $p < 0.01$). If such a convention is used, and it usually is, a result of $p = 0.04$ would be described by the authors as a 'significant' result (in a statistical sense). However, if $p = 0.06$, as this is larger than $p < 0.05$, the latter probability would be described as 'not significant' (at $p < 0.05$). However, as is now obvious there is in fact very little difference between $p = 0.04$ and $p = 0.06$. It is most important to realise that even if the differences in prevalence are 'not significant' they may still be true, but may simply mean that the sample size is not large enough.

The other bit of jargon in the above statement is that a 'two-tailed test' was used. This is because before the survey it was considered that if the prevalence of urinary tract infection differed between the sexes, either sex could have had the higher prevalence. It is often difficult, or controversial, to know when a one-tailed test can be used, but its use in the example given would imply that women have at least as many urinary tract infections as men (either the prevalence is the same, or women have more frequent infections). If a one-tailed test had been used the p value would be half that given.

To calculate the p value various assumptions are made and these are never completely true. If most come close to being true the tests are appropriate, but it usually needs skilled statistical judgement to know when the assumptions are appropriate.

Thus, statistical significance is a question that is frequently asked about health service data and one that should be understood by those concerned. It attempts to sort out whether any differences found are likely to be genuine or simply due to chance. It does not mean that statistically significant results are important, nor is a 'non-significant' result necessarily unimportant. A new piece of apparatus may do a particular test significantly quicker ($p < 0.01$), but if it takes 49 minutes instead of 50 minutes and costs much more, it may well not be desirable.

Measures of Dispersion

'The mean length of stay in hospital after the operation was 10 ± 4 days (s.d.).' The ± 4 days refers to the standard deviation, which is a measure of the spread of the results around the mean of 10 days. One could, of course, give the *range* of the length of stay, from the shortest to the longest, but the disadvantage of the range is that it may give undue prominence to an isolated case. For example, if there was data for 200 cases and 199 had lengths of stay less than 20 days but one patient developed another illness and stayed in hospital for eight weeks, the range would be up to 56 days. This is rather misleading as the next longest length of stay was 19 days. The standard deviation (which should only be used in certain circumstances) is a measure of variation of the results around the mean. The standard deviation is particularly useful if the data are 'normally' distributed. A normal distribution is a particular type of symmetrical distribution about the mean. If the distribution is roughly normal, and again it is best if a statistician judges whether or not this is so, the standard deviation will give an idea of the shape of the distribution (Figure 6.1). Roughly 68 per cent of observations lie within one standard deviation of the mean and 95 per cent of observations lie within two standard deviations of the mean. In the example given above the standard deviation was given as four. As roughly 68 per cent of observations lie within one standard deviation from the mean, one knows that about 68 per cent will have a length of stay between 6 and 14 days, about 2½ per cent will have a length of stay of less than 2 days and about 2½ per cent will have a length of stay of more than 18 days. Of course, if the distribution is not normal these figures, especially the use of the two standard deviations, may not be even roughly correct.

The Accuracy of the Mean

If a mean value is quoted, it is useful to know how accurate this value is thought to be. This is done using a *standard error*. It is calculated by dividing the standard deviation by the square root of the number of observations. If there were 81 observations in the above example the standard error would be written as 10 ± 0.44 (s.e.). Again, assuming a normal distribution, the true mean for the length of stay will in fact lie

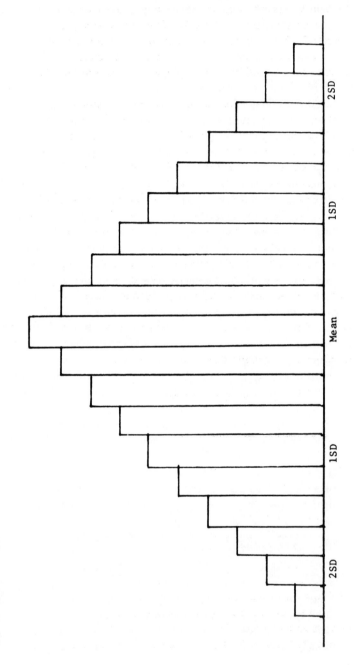

Figure 6.1: A Symmetrical and Roughly Normal Distribution Showing Mean and Standard Deviations (SD = Standard Deviation)

within two standard errors of the mean, that is between 9.12 days and 10.88 days, with approximately 95 per cent confidence.

7 THE EPIDEMIOLOGY OF SOME COMMON DISEASES

7.1. The Epidemiology of Ischaemic Heart Disease

What is Ischaemic Heart Disease?

Ischaemic heart disease is also known as arteriosclerotic heart disease and is usually caused by fatty deposits in the wall of the coronary arteries which reduce the size of the lumen. These deposits can ulcerate and cause thrombi to form on them, which can lead to partial or complete occlusion of the vessel lumen. This may be aggravated by arterial spasm. There are three main clinical presentations of ischaemic heart disease.

Angina, or more specifically *angina pectoris* is chest pain on exertion but relieved by rest, due to chronic narrowing of the coronary arteries. Epidemiologically its prevalence and importance can be studied by means of questionnaires (Rose and Blackburn 1968). *Myocardial infarction* indicates death of cardiac muscle occurring suddenly on previous chronic but sometimes symptomless ischaemic heart disease. In myocardial infarction the pain is typically longer-lasting than in angina pectoris (with a duration of half an hour or more). Some myocardial infarctions occur without symptoms (silent infarcts) but can be recognised by changes in the electrocardiogram, the blood pressure and serum enzyme levels. The third manifestation of ischaemic heart disease, which may follow a history of angina pectoris or myocardial infarction, or may occur 'out of the blue', is *sudden death*. This happens when an infarction causes fatal cardiac arrhythmias. The epidemiology of ischaemic heart disease is reviewed by Tunstall Pedoe (1982: 103) and by the Department of Health and Social Security (1981).

The Importance of Ischaemic Heart Disease

Ischaemic heart disease is one of or the most common cause of death in most economically advanced countries. We have information on this for the British population from the death certificates which are completed by a medical practitioner for each and every death that occurs in this country. The statistics are published annually by the Office of Population Censuses and Surveys. The latest published material relates to 1978 (Table 7.1) which shows that nearly a third of all deaths in males and

64

nearly a quarter of all deaths in females, are due to ischaemic heart disease. In both sexes and at all ages the mortality rate for ischaemic heart disease has shown a marked increase over the last thirty years or so. For men below the age of 50 years, the rate has doubled in the last 20 years alone. This enormous increase, which has rightly been described as a modern epidemic, has fortunately now slowed down and has even halted in certain age groups, especially in men, during the last few years. In women, the rate of increase has been rather less steep than in men, but there is less evidence of any recent improvements in the rates. In some countries of the world, and in particular in the United States, there has been a recent decrease, since the 1960s, from the very high rates of mortality from ischaemic heart disease. The exact reasons for the great increase, and now the slight decrease, in mortality from this condition are still not entirely understood. In many developing countries mortality rates are rising fast. Some of the changes in the *number* of deaths in England and Wales can be explained by changes in the age structure of the population. The mortality rate from this condition increases very greatly with age.

Table 7.1: England and Wales 1978: Mortality from Ischaemic Heart Disease (IHD)

	Death from IHD	Death from all causes
Males	92,380 (31.3%)	295,505
Females	68,078 (23.4%)	290,396

Source: *OPCS Mortality Statistics* 1978 (Published 1980).

Table 7.2 shows that the mortality rate in men aged 75 and over is more than a hundred times the rate in men who are aged between 25 and 44 years. In women the rate of increase with age is even more marked. From this it follows that in the younger age groups there is an enormous sex difference in mortality from ischaemic heart disease. Table 7.2 shows that in the age group 25-44 years the rate in men is more than six times the rate in women. However, for those aged 75 years and over the rate in women is about two-thirds the rate in men. Even in those aged over 85 years, the death rates from ischaemic heart disease are still higher in men than in women.

Table 7.2: England and Wales 1978: Mortality from Ischaemic Heart Disease by Age per 100,000 Population

	25-44	45-64	65-74	75 and over
Males	31	498	1,669	3,533
Females	5	128	696	2,323

Source: *OPCS Mortality Statistics* 1978 (Published 1980).

As well as the changes that have occurred in the age structure of the population there must be other important factors determining the changes in mortality. It is obvious that the changes in mortality could be due to two quite separate factors, or a combination of these two factors. The first factor is the incidence of ischaemic heart disease in the population, that is the number developing the disease. The second possible factor is the mortality rate amongst those who have the condition. It is likely that changes in treatment have had some effect on mortality, however, it is remarkably difficult to get good evidence on the evaluation of treatment of acute attacks of this disease. However, the evidence indicates that probably the major cause of the increase (and now possibly the decrease) in mortality from ischaemic heart disease has been changes in the incidence of the disease. We must regard this conclusion also as somewhat tentative, however, because, surprisingly, there is very little information anywhere in the world about the changes in the incidence of this disease. A great number of individual surveys have been done which have measured the incidence and prevalence of ischaemic heart disease in certain populations over a short period of time. Disappointingly, there is virtually no information about how this rate has changed over a period of ten years or more. If this statement causes some surprise, it must be remembered that many cases of ischaemic heart disease are not admitted to hospital. For this reason it is not appropriate to use the routine hospital statistics to look at the changes in incidence of this disease over a period of time. Obviously many of the less severe cases of ischaemic heart disease may be treated at home. However, as already mentioned, mortality from ischaemic heart disease can be sudden and some deaths occur with no prior warning. The statistics for 1978, for example, show that of the 92,380 deaths in males, 39,513 occurred at home — this is nearly 43 per cent of all the deaths from this disease. Death occurred neither in hospital nor at home in 12,585 men. Presumably these are largely deaths occurring at work, in the street and elsewhere. While we have a considerable amount of information on the deaths, we know much less about those who have the disease and survive.

Geographical Variations in Mortality

There are great differences in the death rates from ischaemic heart disease in various countries of the world, with Finland, Northern Ireland and Scotland having the highest rates. These rates are nearly ten times those of Japan. Even within England and Wales there are considerable differences between the highest and the lowest death rates for ischaemic heart disease, such that the rates are about twice as high in some areas as they are in others. There is a general tendency for the mortality rates to be lower in the south and east of England and higher in the north and west. None of these differences is explained by the age structure of these populations. Within Britain, there appears to be no consistent urban/rural difference in the mortality from this condition but there is an increased mortality in the winter months, especially during periods of extreme cold.

Risk Factors for Ischaemic Heart Disease

A number of epidemiological studies have looked at risk factors for ischaemic heart disease, and it has been shown that it is possible to identify people who are at higher risk of developing this disease. The greatest risk factor, which has already been mentioned, is the age of the individual, as in both sexes the risk increases markedly with increasing age. There is also the sex difference, which is particularly important in the younger age groups, but men continue to have a higher risk than women right up to extreme old age. Other known risk factors are listed in Table 7.3.

Table 7.3: Risk Factors for Ischaemic Heart Disease

1. Age
2. Sex
3. Smoking
4. Blood pressure
5. Diet
6. Diabetes mellitus
7. Family history
8. Contraceptive pill
9. Lack of physical activity
10. Stress/personality
11. Soft water

In the past, cigarette smoking has been particularly associated in the public mind with the greatly increased risks of lung cancer and chronic bronchitis. However, an examination of the deaths that are associated with smoking shows that at least half are in fact due to cardiovascular disease. It has been estimated that for men between the ages of 45 and 54, smoking more than 40 cigarettes a day increases the chances of dying from ischaemic heart disease by a factor of ten, compared with non-smokers of a similar age. Smoking 10-20 cigarettes per day increases the chances of dying by a factor of six, again compared with non-smokers.

Numerous studies have shown the association between a rise in arterial blood pressure, whether systolic or diastolic, and an increased risk of ischaemic heart disease. This increase in risk seems to be gradual and progressive, with increasing levels of blood pressure. Even individuals with quite modestly raised blood pressures, for example a systolic pressure of 130 mmHg, carry a slightly higher risk. Again, to take the example of men between the ages of 45 and 54 years, a systolic pressure of 180 mmHg increases the chances of developing ischaemic heart disease by about three times. However, although those individuals with very high levels of blood pressure are at greatest risk, the largest number of episodes of ischaemic heart disease occur in those with only moderately raised levels of blood pressure. This apparent anomaly is simply due to the fact that in the general population there are very large numbers of individuals with only slightly raised blood pressure levels. Although the risk to any individual in this group is relatively slight, because of the large number of people involved many of the cases do occur in this group. Although the rate is higher in those with higher blood pressures, the number of individuals with extremely high levels of blood pressure is sufficiently few to make this a relatively small contribution to the total number of cases occurring in a community. From the point of view of trying to reduce the incidence of ischaemic heart disease, this therefore means that large numbers of individuals have to have their blood pressure lowered in order for there to be a substantial beneficial effect in the population as a whole.

The contribution of diet to the incidence of ischaemic heart disease is more controversial than is the contribution of both smoking and blood pressure. Undoubtedly those individuals with a high plasma cholesterol level are at higher risk. The situation is made rather more complicated, as only rather over 10 per cent of the total body cholesterol is in the plasma and studies have shown that the plasma level is a rather poor indicator of the total body lipids. Another measurement which is sometimes made is the plasma level of triglycerides. In a report of a joint working group of the Royal College of Physicians of London and the

British Cardiac Society (1976) it was recommended that there should not be widespread population screening for plasma lipid levels, although certain groups at high risk, with strong family histories of ischaemic heart disease or familial hypercholesterolaemia, should be tested. The working party, however, recommended that there should be a general reduction in the amount of fats (towards 35 per cent of total calories in the diet) and that there should be a partial substitution of saturated fats (largely from animals and dairy products but also some hard margarines and lard) by polyunsaturated fats (such as corn oil and sunflower oil). Another aspect of diet which has been widely researched in the past is the role of sugar, however many studies in this country have now suggested that variation in sugar intake is unlikely to be an important part of the cause of ischaemic heart disease. In recent years there has also been great interest shown in the part played by dietary fibre in prevention of numerous diseases, including ischaemic heart disease. The importance of dietary fibre is still controversial but the working party recommended individuals to eat more vegetables and fruit of all kinds.

Two other controversial aspects of diet concern the finding of some investigations that coffee-drinking may be associated with a higher risk of ischaemic heart disease, and that salt intake may also be important, particularly with regard to the development of hypertension. A number of studies have now suggested that a modest intake of alcohol may reduce the incidence of ischaemic heart disease, but this has not been evaluated by means of a randomised clinical trial! There is good evidence that in areas where the drinking water is hard, the mortality from ischaemic heart disease is rather lower than would otherwise be expected. It is likely that obesity, from whatever cause, is a factor in the incidence of ischaemic heart disease. However, several epidemiological surveys have suggested that obesity, in itself, contributes relatively little to the onset of ischaemic heart disease, but they do confirm that obesity is often associated with other features of increased risk (e.g. plasma lipids and high blood pressure). Obesity may, therefore, be a useful overall index of risk and is particularly valuable as it is easy to pick out such individuals without detailed screening tests.

The presence of diabetes mellitus or a family history of ischaemic heart disease increases the chances of an individual developing the disease. There is now much evidence that women on the contraceptive pill have a higher risk of developing ischaemic heart disease; whether this risk is important or not depends largely upon the presence of other risk factors. In younger women with normal blood pressures and normal plasma lipids, who are non-smokers, although the risk may be increased, it is already so low as to be almost non-existent. However, in women over the age of 35 years, especially those who have other risk factors, taking the contraceptive pill may increase the risk of their developing ischaemic heart disease to an unjustifiable extent.

The protective effect of physical exercise has for some time been a controversial issue, though in general those who take more exercise have lower risks of ischaemic heart disease. The question still remains as to how often this is cause and effect; is it the physical activity in itself that is reducing the risk of ischaemic heart disease, or is it that those people who take part in physical activities are also likely to be non-smokers and to eat balanced diets? It is always difficult, when comparing those who do a considerable amount of physical activity with those who are less active, to be certain that one is comparing otherwise similar groups. However, a number of the more recent studies do strongly suggest that physical activity in itself may be protective against ischaemic heart disease.

Stress and personality are two more controversial risk factors for ischaemic heart disease. One of the difficulties is how one can measure stress and personality and also how to bring about a beneficial change in individual cases. There has been an interesting change in mortality in the different social classes; originally ischaemic heart disease was more frequent in social classes I and II and was linked with an executive life style, however, more recently this has changed and now mortality is higher in manual workers.

Reduction of Mortality in Ischaemic Heart Disease

In view of the fact that most deaths from ischaemic heart disease take place outside hospital, and because most of the deaths that occurred within the first month took place within one hour of the onset of the symptoms, it is very unlikely that more effective hospital treatment could substantially reduce the mortality in the community from ischaemic heart disease. There are two other lines of approach. Firstly, there is the education and training of individuals in the community to understand the appropriate first aid and treatment which can be applied at once when individuals suffer their attack. This immediate first aid can then be backed up by a fast and efficient cardiac ambulance service. This method of approach, trying to reduce the immediate mortality, has been adopted in some cities but, however effective, it will not prevent the numerous cases in which death is sudden. Therefore, the main approach to reducing mortality from ischaemic heart disease must be to try and prevent the disease altogether. This can be done by taking the various factors mentioned in Table 7.3 and seeing which can be changed to reduce the risk. Age cannot, and sex can very rarely, be changed! Little can be done in those with a family history or diabetes except to reduce other risk factors with particular vigour, even then the results in diabetics have been rather disappointing. The best hope at present is reducing the amount of smoking, especially cigarette smoking, reducing blood pressure levels by drugs and other means, and encouraging balanced diets and sensible physical activity.

7.2 Epidemiology of Renal Disease

Mortality statistics give two major groups of deaths from kidney disease. The first of these is infections of the kidney and the second is nephritis and nephrosis. In a patient dying from end-stage kidney disease the distinction between the different diseases is sometimes difficult. In the 1950s the introduction of the concept of *significant bacteriuria*, and the widespread availability of new broad-spectrum antibiotics, produced hope that the mortality from infections of the kidney would fall. However, an analysis of the mortality statistics suggests that not only was this not so, but that in fact the number of deaths ascribed to infections of the kidney was actually rising. No logical interpretation of this trend was apparent, but it was noted that the increase in the mortality from infections of the kidney was being paralleled by a decrease in the mortality from other causes of kidney failure. This is shown in Figure 7.1. It will be noted that this is a gradual change and therefore a reclassification of the causes of death, which is carried out every now and again, does not seem to be the explanation. As the increase in mortality from infections of the kidney and a decrease in mortality from nephritis and nephrosis occurred in both sexes and in all age groups, it is likely that this was a change in diagnostic fashion on the part of doctors writing the death certificates, rather than a real change in the mortality from these two groups of diseases (Figure 7.2). While the latter cannot be ruled out, the chances of it happening in both sexes and in all age groups, so that the decline in one disease is similar to the increase in the other, seems very remote. Although Figure 7.1, based on numbers, shows no evidence of a decline in mortality, Figure 7.2, based on age-specific death rates, does show evidence of an overall decline in all groups except the oldest group of women. This real change has been missed in Figure 7.1 which took no account of changes in the number of women in the population nor of changes in the age structure of the population.

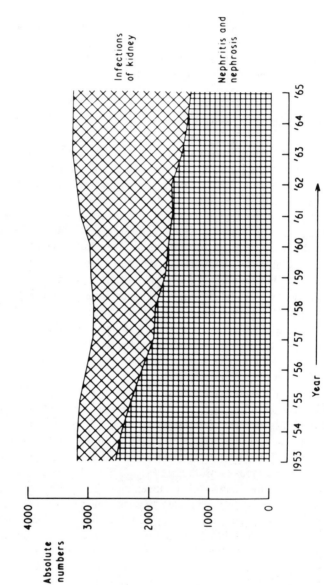

Figure 7.1: Number of Deaths from Nephritis and Nephrosis (I.C.D. 590-4) and Infections of Kidney (I.C.D. 600) in Females in England and Wales 1953-65

Figure 7.2: Death Rates for Nephritis and Nephrosis (I.C.D. 590-4) and Infections of Kidney (I.C.D. 600) in Four Age Groups in England and Wales 1953-65

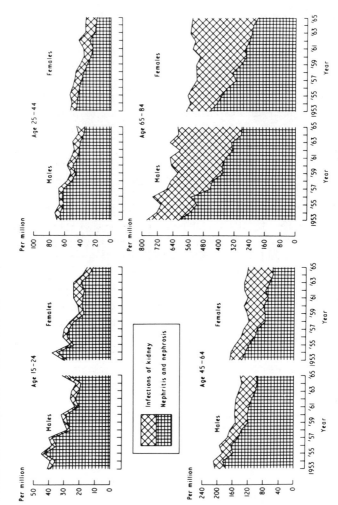

The most likely explanation for the events described above is that the introduction of the concept of significant bacteruria and the availability of broad-spectrum antibiotics resulted in more intense investigation of patients with kidney disease, and in particular a search for those with evidence of infection. This would have been attempted in view of the broad-spectrum antibiotics which offered the hope of more efficacious treatment.

The Treatment of End-term Kidney Failure

Although the number of patients with treatable chronic kidney failure in Britain is relatively small, it poses a most striking problem in the allocation of resources and in the provision of life-saving treatment for this minority of patients. It is thought that the number of people below the age of 60 years who are suitable for this treatment is roughly 40 per million of the population per year. During the 1960s rapid advances were made in the treatment of kidney failure by dialysis. This resulted in a technique, which had previously been suitable only for treatment of acute short-term renal failure, becoming suitable for long-term treatment. Also, about the same time and because of the introduction of immunosuppressive drugs, it was possible to transplant kidneys from one person into another, or from a cadaver into a living patient. Earlier the only successful kidney operations were done on identical twins, who do not have the same immunological problems of rejection. During the last 20 years considerable progress has been made in both the dialysis of patients and transplantation of kidneys. Both methods of treatment, often of course used in combination, provide life-saving treatment for many patients with kidney disease. However, the technology for the treatment of these patients developed much faster than the resources of the National Health Service could provide facilities. To be fair this situation arose not only in Britain but in most countries of the world. Indeed, in the 1960s and early 1970s Britain was treating a higher proportion of its cases of kidney failure than most other countries. In the early 1970s three studies in Wales, Scotland and Northern Ireland set out to look at the incidence of chronic renal failure. This was found to be about 40-50 per million of total population per year who were judged to be suitable for dialysis and/or transplantation, and who were under 60 or 65 years of age. As facilities for treating these people were not always available, it was up to individual clinicians to make decisions about which patients could be treated and which patients would not be accepted for a treatment which would reduce their chances of dying very considerably (Office of Health Economics report No. 62, 1978).

Extremely good statistical material on the number of patients treated for kidney failure throughout Europe is available from data regularly published by the European Dialysis and Transplant Association (EDTA). The figure of 40 per million total population given above as the incidence of treatable kidney failure will produce a considerable number of patients on kidney treatment over the years, as this incidence figure is the number of new cases developing each year. The more efficacious the treatment is, and the lower the mortality in those receiving treatment, the larger will be the accumulated number of patients on treatment for kidney failure. If dialysis is the treatment this will need to be continued on a regular basis. If a transplant is the treatment then the patient may need relatively little management once the initial stage of the operation is over. However, not all transplants last for more than a few years, and therefore it is likely that many patients who are treated by a transplant may require dialysis when the transplant fails, with a possibility of a further transplant being required at a later stage. There is a further difficulty in providing treatment for all who might benefit as with increasing sophistication in the techniques, it is possible that a number of patients who would previously have been considered unsuitable, either because of their age or because of other diseases which co-exist, may now be amenable to successful treatment for their kidney failure. Allowing for these trends, and assuming that the life expectation of people being accepted for dialysis and transplantation would be nearly similar to that of other individuals of the same age, it has been calculated that it might become necessary to treat about 1000 patients per million of the population. This is many, many times greater than are treated by the existing facilities (Office of Health Economics report No. 62, 1978).

We thus have an example of a relatively expensive yet efficacious form of treatment that is not widely available to all who might benefit, despite the existence of the National Health Service. The fact that some of the initial units for dialysis and transplantation were centrally funded allowed Britain to become one of the best providers of these methods of treatment in their early stages of development. However, since the 1974 reorganisation of the National Health Service, the provision of resources has been decided at a local level, and it is during this time, in the absence of strong leadership from the DHSS, that Britain has fallen behind many other Western European countries in the availability of provision for treating kidney disease.

Allocation of Scarce Resources

It is possible to consider the allocation of scarce resources, such as those used to treat patients in chronic renal failure, in three categories. The first and most obvious one is the rationing of the service, which is available in the free market, by a fee. The second category, which is called *implicit rationing*, is that currently in existence in Britain (Office of Health Economics report No. 64, 1979). Here the individual clinicians in practice have to use rationing because they see more patients than there are facilities to treat. This is particularly distressful for the clinicians concerned, especially as many other treatments, which have been far less validated, are available to patients under the National Health Service without such rationing. This situation has arisen, as described above, because of the very rapid changes in technology over the last quarter of a century and, in virtually all countries of the world, the slow response of those organising medical care to make provision to treat all patients who would benefit. However, if one rejects the free market solution to this problem, the only alternative to implicit rationing is *explicit rationing*, where 'guidelines' would be issued for clinicians to follow when making decisions on which patients should, and which should not, receive treatment. This is a bureaucratic solution to the problem, and one that is generally unacceptable to health professionals; it would be associated with a very rigid attitude to the problem of caring for those dying of kidney disease and may be very difficult to develop in the future. However, in the United States it has been accepted that such treatments, because they are so efficacious, should be made available to all. As long ago as 1972 the Senate voted to extend medicare coverage for chronic renal failure, so that it should apply to almost the entire population. This was seen as a step towards comprehensive national insurance against 'catastrophic' illness in the United States. It is also a good example of the way that the method of financing arrangements can affect not only the amount of treatment available but also the type and place of treatment, as the administrative arrangements discourage transplantation and very much favour dialysis in centres rather than at home (Office of Health Economics report No. 62, 1978).

There is one other concept of rationing which should be mentioned which has been known as 'rationing by science'. This is based on the fact that when scientific evaluation has shown that certain treatments are efficacious they should be applied to all who might benefit. Resources for doing this should come, if necessary, from those presently being used for other treatments in which the evidence of their efficaciousness is more limited or non-existent. This theory has been argued by Cochrane (1971) who stresses that if unnecessary treatments could be eliminated, the resources already devoted to the Health Service would be sufficient to meet all the scientifically proven needs. Surely on this basis, the treatment of kidney failure would be extended to many who do not now receive its undoubted benefits?

7.3 Home Accidents

Home accidents can be considered in terms of their epidemiological investigation in the same way as any other disease; accidents are classified as diseases within the World Health Organisation (1978). Fatal home accidents accounted for approximately one per cent of deaths from all causes in England and Wales in 1979, and approximately one-third of all deaths from accidents of all causes (Table 7.4). Non-fatal home accidents account for approximately 20 per cent of all attendances at accident and emergency units, as found in a study by Cliff (1973: 4-7) amongst patients attending eight major accident and emergency units.

Table 7.4: England and Wales 1979: Deaths from Selected Causes of Accidents and Violence

Cause	Number	Proportion
Road Transport	5,865	28%
Home	5,739	27%
Other Causes	9,549	45%
All Causes	21,153	100%

Source: Office of Population Censuses and Surveys *Mortality Statistics Accidents and Violence 1979* (England and Wales), Table 1, p. 6.

The World Health Organisation defined an accident as 'an unpredetermined event resulting in a recognisable injury', and in this section home accidents will be confined to those that resulted in a recognisable injury.

Most of the information relating to home accidents comes either from mortality or morbidity data, the latter mainly obtained from hospital statistics, since there is no routine source of data relating to those injury accidents attending a general practitioner. Thus, the current statistical information about home accidents will not necessarily reflect the true picture, but is of sufficient value to provide the epidemiologist with information to ascertain the distribution and determinants of these accidents.

Whilst much of our knowledge about home accidents has had to come from studies of fatal home accidents, more data is now becoming routinely available on non-fatal accidents. This has been due in part to the introduction in 1977 by the then Department of Prices and Consumer Protection (now the Department of Trade) of an ongoing study in a sample of hospital accident and emergency units throughout England and Wales. In these units patients who attended as a result of a home accident were asked to co-operate in the study and provide additional information about the nature and cause of their accident. In addition, a number of *ad hoc* studies have been carried out into the problems of home accidents, and these have included studies by Backett (1965), Cargill (1967) and Goulding (1978: 91-5). In investigating the epidemiology of home accidents most investigators have adopted the simple technique of examining the problem under the headings of who?, where?, when? and why? Using this approach, the investigators can gain information about a range of factors which may be involved in the aetiology of a particular type of accident in the home and in this chapter this approach will be adopted to illustrate the investigation of home accidents.

Who?

The age-specific mortality from fatal home accidents in England and Wales in 1979 per million of the population is illustrated in Table 7.5. The table shows the age groups who are principally 'at risk' from fatal home accidents. These principally involve children under the age of one, children aged 1-4 years and the elderly, particularly those aged 75 years and over. The table indicates also that from the age of 45 years onwards there is an increasing risk of home accidents in both males and females and, whilst in the earlier years males have a higher mortality rate, in the age group 75 years and over females have nearly twice the mortality rate compared to males. This simple type of analysis helps to identify the age groups where further investigation is needed into the factors which may be associated with this high mortality.

Table 7.5: England and Wales 1979: Deaths from Accidents in the Home and Residential Institutions by Age Groups and Sex per Million Population

Sex	< 1	1-4	5-14	15-44	45-64	65-74	75+	All Ages
Males	252	57	16	40	78	187	876	91
Females	200	45	8	24	72	187	1224	141

Source: Office of Population Censuses and Surveys *Mortality Statistics Accidents and Violence 1979* (England and Wales) Table 5, p. 25.

Analysis of morbidity data from the Department of Prices and Consumer Protection's Report (1977: 4) shows a quite different picture and this is illustrated in Table 7.6. The table illustrates that in terms of the proportion of people attending hospital accident and emergency units for treatment of non-fatal home accidents, 44 per cent were aged 0-14 years, but only 6 per cent were aged 75 years and over. Care must be taken, however, in interpreting this data since it is not a rate, that is the numbers are not related to the population at risk. The data only refers to the proportion of people in the various age groups who attended for care, this being a proportional analysis. The evidence, however, suggests that in terms of mortality the very young and the very old are principally at risk, but for non-fatal accidents the very young, and in particular those aged 0-4 years, are principally at risk.

Table 7.6: England and Wales 1977: Proportion of Attendance at Accident and Emergency Units by Age Groups and Sex, Jan-June 1977, as a Result of a Home Accident

Sex	0-4	5-14	15-29	30-44	45-64	65-74	75+	Not Known
Males	14.5	10.5	8.0	5.8	4.9	1.7	1.1	0.1
Females	10.7	8.3	9.3	7.2	8.7	3.9	4.9	0.1
Total	25.3	18.9	17.3	13.0	13.6	5.6	6.1	0.2

Source: Department of Prices and Consumer Protection *The Home Accident Surveillance System 1977* (England and Wales), Table 1, p. 4.

When?

Under this heading the epidemiologist is looking for trends over time and these may relate to seasonal variations, times of the week or times of the day. Data from the Office of Population Censuses and Surveys (1981: 11) suggests that there are seasonal variations in mortality from home accidents, the months of November to March inclusive showing a higher number of fatal accidents compared to the spring and summer months. Some caution has to be expressed because again these are whole numbers and do not relate to the population at risk, but if a crude mortality rate is calculated, using the total population at risk, then there does appear to be a seasonal variation in the fatal home accident rates. Evidence from the Department of Prices and Consumer Protection Study (1976: 11) indicated that there were slight variations in the proportion of people attending accident and emergency units with home accidents on Sundays and Mondays, but this was not a statistically significant difference from other days of the week.

Hancock (1973: 77-80) in a study of children brought to the accident and emergency unit of the Children's Hospital in Sheffield, found that 15 per cent of the child poisonings occurred during the period 0800-0900 and 27 per cent between 1700-2000 hours. Both times correspond to maximal family activity, when observation of all children would be difficult. Thus, from this type of investigation it is possible to identify periods, not only during the day or week, but even within the year, when various age groups may be more at risk than others and when accidents in the home are more likely to occur. In a more recent analysis of the data from the Home Accident Surveillance System under the Department of Trade (1981: 28-31) non-fatal home accidents were shown to have a marked peak during the month of May and again during the months of July and August. Further analysis of this data indicates that a high proportion of these are related to outdoor accidents, and that during May, June and August the garden, or grassed areas adjacent to the home, are the site for many of these home accidents. This type of information is important in the context of the prevention of accidents, but also illustrates the problem of surveillance of children by parents, particularly during the holiday periods.

Where?

In the epidemiological investigation of home accidents, statistically the information is related to two identifiable living units. These are: the home (referring to domestic living premises and the areas adjacent to them, e.g. gardens, pathways); residential institutions (referring to institutions which include boarding schools, hospitals, nursing homes and old people's homes, where a person is temporarily or permanently resident). This is an important distinction because the two types of living units have clearly identifiable different populations. In residential institutions the population will be predominantly elderly whereas in the home a population is very much more varied and is representative of the general population of England and Wales. In addition, residential institutions may not only have a high proportion of elderly but also infirm people, that is their population is not representative of the general population.

From mortality data provided by the Office of Population Censuses and Surveys (1981: 12-24) it is possible to identify where certain home accidents occurred. This can include not only whether it was in a private dwelling, but whether it involved a fall from ladders, scaffolding, falls from one level to another and whether fire was involved. Using morbidity data from the Department of Prices and Consumer Protection Report

(1977: 7) an analysis of the location of non-fatal accidents in the home was presented. Of non-fatal accidents 16 per cent occurred in the kitchen, 16 per cent in the living-dining area, 11 per cent in the garden, 9 per cent on inside stairs and 8 per cent in bedrooms. Data from the Department of Trade (1981: 18) indicated there had been little change from the previous findings, and that the kitchen and living-dining area were still the most common areas where home accidents occurred. Thus, by investigating where the accident occurs it is possible to identify particular areas in the home which are potentially 'at risk' locations, and thus where there is a need to identify the cause and possibly preventive measures.

Why?

The causal factors of home accidents can be grouped for statistical purposes under five main headings, poisonings, falls, burns, choking and suffocation, and all other causes. Table 7.7 analyses the four major groups in terms of their mortality rate per million by age and sex for England and Wales in 1979. This analysis of the major causes of home accidents identifies that falls are one of the most prominent causes of fatal accidents. The analysis also indicates the different accident rates for the four main causes, highlighting specific age groups where there is concern.

Table 7.7: England and Wales 1979: Home Accidents: Deaths per Million by Age Group and Selected Causes

| | Cause and Sex | | | | | | | |
| | Poisoning | | Falls | | Burns | | Suffocation* | |
Age Group (years)	M	F	M	F	M	F	M	F
Under 1	3	—	6	3	6	20	189	143
1 - 4	2	3	8	4	22	14	9	14
5 - 14	—	—	2	1	4	4	7	1
15 - 44	12	9	7	4	5	5	7	3
45 - 64	10	18	31	24	13	11	11	8
65 - 74	10	14	102	109	29	25	18	16
75+	11	11	635	986	94	105	31	30

* Includes accidental suffocation and choking.
Source: Office of Population Censuses and Surveys, *Mortality Statistics Accidents and Violence 1979* (England and Wales), Table 5, pp. 25-6.

Within each of the groupings identified in the table, special studies have been carried out to investigate whether there are any particular factors contributing to both mortality and morbidity. In a study by

Smith (1976: 1872-6) he found that trips, drops and hypotensive attacks were identified as being associated with falls, particularly in the elderly. A study of factors involved in poisonings had indicated that there has been a marked decline in mortality from poisonings due to domestic gas supplies. Alphey and Leach (1974: 97-102) showed that the change from coal gas to North Sea (natural) gas had been a major factor in reducing accidental poisoning from this cause. Table 7.8 shows the decline in mortality from domestic gas poisoning between 1964 and 1979.

Table 7.8: England and Wales: Home Accidents Resulting from Accidental Poisoning from Domestic Gas Supplies 1964 and 1979

Deaths	1964	1979
Total	935	84
Male	395	45
Female	540	39

Sources: (1) General Register Office, *Registrar General's Statistical Review 1964* (England and Wales), Table 7, p. 35; (2) Office of Population Censuses and Surveys, *Mortality Statistics Accidents and Violence 1979* (England and Wales), Table 4, p. 14.

Studies of mortality and morbidity data provide epidemiologists and those concerned with the prevention of accidents with information about the cause and the factors involved. This is of particular importance to nurses in general, and health visitors and district nurses in particular, because the latter have access to people's homes. In addition, health education officers and social workers should be aware of the information that can be obtained by epidemiological studies in order that this can provide new thoughts on advice about prevention of accidents in the home.

Community nurses have a particularly important part to play in identifying causes of home accidents and suggesting ways of reducing the risks and hence the prevention of accidents. In looking for simple factors the simple methodological approach could be adopted, which is summarised as follows:

(1)   Identify the user — is she/he able to use the equipment and cope with the environment?
(2)   Identify the equipment — is it safe, does the user know how to use it and is it suitable for the environment?
(3)   Identify the environment — is it as safe as it should be?

Using this type of methodology it is possible to identify where the main causes of concern could be within a particular household. Even if an accident has occurred and treatment has been sought in the accident and emergency unit there is still an opportunity for nurses to be involved in the epidemiological study of these accidents. In discussion with the patients it is possible to identify where the accident occurred, and perhaps to give advice on how to prevent accidents in the future. Thus, accident and emergency departments can be a prime source of epidemiological information about home accidents and carefully taken histories of the cause are important in the study of the aetiology and prevention.

Epidemiological investigations of home accidents can provide information about the distribution and determinants of these accidents. Determination of the cause is an essential feature in prevention for it provides information to the nursing profession, who have access to people in their homes, as well as to health education staff, as to the main and potential areas to which particular attention needs to be paid. In a recent study undertaken in the University of Southampton's Community Medicine Department (1982) parents whose children had suffered a home accident were asked to identify where they thought the most dangerous place was in the home. Analysis of the replies indicated that the kitchen, stairs and bathroom-toilet were the areas which parents thought were most dangerous to children. The replies, therefore, suggested that they did not consider the living-dining area as a potentially dangerous place. This is important information since the evidence already quoted has shown that the living-dining area, with the kitchen, is one of the most common locations for a home accident. Thus, in the investigation of home accidents it is important not only to examine the evidence from the medical point of view but also to identify parents' perception of areas of danger in the home, as these may conflict with the medical findings, as illustrated in the Southampton study.

Home accidents continue to present a challenge in terms of accident prevention, being one of the commonest causes of accidents and causing a similar number of deaths per annum as road accidents. Road accidents receive a great deal of publicity and large sums of money are spent on preventive measures, but similar expenditure does not occur in respect of home accidents.

Prevention of home accidents involves not only education, but engineering for safe products and also legislation. In respect of the latter the Department of Trade is responsible for ensuring that agreements made with manufacturers in respect of products are maintained and meet British standards. Such legislation under the Consumer Protection Act has covered the manufacture of oil heaters, such that when they tip more than 45° the flame is automatically extinguished. This legislation was introduced in 1962, followed in 1966 by further legislation. Other legislation has covered such items as nightdresses, electric appliances, electric blankets, cooking utensils, heating appliances, pencils and graphic instruments (related to lead content) and children's clothing, with specific relation to hood cords. This legislation and the engineering that has taken place to improve safety has unfortunately always been as a result of fatal accidents, but there is evidence of closer involvement between many agencies and the medical profession in respect of designing safer homes for children, as indicated in the book edited by Jackson (1977).

Community nurses have a particularly important role to play in the prevention of home accidents; their access to the home gives them a unique opportunity for intimate observation of the family. Health visitors have a special function through their training in prevention. In addition, however, hospital-based nurses working particularly in the accident and emergency units, but also in the ward situation, can also play a helpful and valuable role in giving advice to those who have been injured in a home accident and perhaps ensuring that they obtain information, either directly from the department itself or through the health visitor or health education service, about possible preventive measures.

7.4 The Epidemiology of Psychiatric Illness

Introduction

In this section the role of epidemiology will be briefly discussed and illustrated in relation to the cause and distribution of psychiatric illness; and the use of epidemiological studies in the planning of psychiatric services. Unlike other illnesses, psychiatric illnesses present greater problems to those who study them since they do not necessarily present with easily-defined symptoms or identifiable pathological consequences (which for some diseases can be measured by changes in blood chemistry), and may be also affected by social and cultural factors. Thus, some psychiatric illnesses present a multifactorial aetiology and the epidemiologist tries to arrive at reliable measures of the incidence and prevalence of these illnesses and to relate these rates to the different factors in the composition and the social and cultural aspects in the population under study (Ashton 1980: 12-16).

As with any epidemiological study, care has to be taken in relating the findings to the population under study. For example, Frerichs,

Aneshensel and Clark (1981: 691-9), examined the prevalence of depression in Los Angeles county in the United States of America. In their study they found a variation amongst the sub-groups of that population in relation to the prevalence of depression. People of Spanish origin had the highest prevalence rates, whilst those termed 'white' had the lowest. Such findings must, however, be taken in the context of the social and economic factors which may also play a part in determining the incidence and prevalence of the disease as suggested by Ashton (1980). When these factors were added to the study in Los Angeles then poverty and educational attainment were significant factors in those who were depressed.

Factors other than socio-economic and cultural have been identified of importance in psychiatric illness. An early study by Davenport and Muncey (1916: 195-222) into Huntington's chorea in New England (USA) showed that genetic factors were involved in the development and spread of this illness in the community. By careful study they were able to retrace the spread of this disease and show that four families could be identified who in the past were probably responsible for the origin of this illness. Their study by careful examination of who, where and when, was able to answer the question why, indicating a hereditary factor.

Other community studies have been able to examine the prevalence of mental subnormality. Cooper and Morgan (1973: 20-3) quote the work of Lewis, who carried out a study in six different locations in England and Wales in 1929. The study was thought to be representative of the whole population of England and Wales and suggested that there might be two groups of mentally subnormal people in the population: those in whom there was an organic cause, and those which were associated with socio-economic factors. Later work, however, indicated that the division in relation to the socio-economic factors was not quite as simple and that organic and socio-economic factors were probably interrelated. These early studies, however, highlighted that there were certain problems in the epidemiological studies into the cause of psychiatric illness and its distribution in the population.

Problems in the Study of Cause and Distribution of Psychiatric Illness

In the introduction attention was drawn to the multifactorial nature of some psychiatric illnesses and this has led to problems of agreement about the criteria for diagnosis and how much social, cultural and economic factors should be involved, and to what extent the illnesses are of organic origin. Some of the practical problems in the study of the cause and distribution of psychiatric illness are outlined below.

Choice of Study.   The choice of the type of study must be appropriate
to the answers being sought. Studies such as those outlined in Chapter 4
can be used to try and determine the cause and distribution of psychiatric illness. In making this choice advice should be sought from a statistician, particularly if sampling is going to be undertaken and, again, this
has been discussed in Chapter 5. Thus, the study of psychiatric illness by
epidemiological studies is determined as for any other illness (disease)
by the question to be answered.

Definition of the Population.   For any study definition of the population is important. This has been outlined in Chapter 5, in relation to
sampling. In studies of psychiatric illness the definition of the population is particularly important, because past studies have shown that
migration due to psychiatric illness does occur, so that the prevalence
of a disease may be lower than expected. This requires careful follow-
up of the population as defined and may require longitudinal studies
of that population, even if some of the population has migrated into
another area. Thus, it is important to ensure, as for other epidemiological studies, that the population is kept as intact as possible.

Case Definition.   There are particular problems in the study of psychiatric illness in terms of case definitions and it is necessary when assessing the value of the study to be aware of the criteria being used and
whether these were, or are, compatible with other study definitions.
For example, Ashton (1980: 25) discussing depression, indicates that
there is confusion in respect of the classification of this illness, partly
due to ambiguous labels used to describe the illness as well as arguments
as to what effect social and cultural factors play. He indicates that there
is still discussion between psychiatrists in an attempt to clarify what
has become an ambiguous situation and suggests that in fact epidemiological studies may not have helped, because psychiatrists are now
'locked in arguments over statistical analyses'.

Case definition relies, however, on individuals in the population
recognising that they have an illness for which help is needed. Surveys
of psychiatric illness encounter the problem of actual illness-recognition
by individuals, in a population which in turn is governed by socio-
cultural factors as to whether the individual will seek help. Kasl and
Cobb (1966: 246-66) suggest that one of the basic problems in illness
behaviour, and hence our understanding of disease, is: in the presence

of symptoms, what will the individual do and why will he do it? Thus, the self-referral of an individual for care is important, since the case definition will of necessity be built up of symptoms presented by individuals to doctors. The reporting of these symptoms may, therefore, become part of the case definition. Case definition needs to be as precise and unambiguous as possible and this is the basis of case-finding and case-identification.

Case-finding and Identification.   This falls into two parts, namely the identification of all known cases and the identification of ill people who are, as yet, unknown to the health care agencies. These are both dependent upon case definition and, as Cooper and Morgan (1973: 38) indicated, in psychiatry the situation is complicated by poor standards of diagnostic reliability and confusion over the boundaries between normality and abnormality.

Identification of Known Cases.   This depends on the availability of morbidity data. Attention has been drawn to the limitations of hospital-based data, where the person concerned is sufficiently disturbed to require hospital admission. Providing resources are adequate for any given population, then there is the possibility that, for certain conditions (such as schizophrenia), all patients will, at some time, come to hospital and hospital admission rates could equate to the incidence and prevalence of the disease. This was a factor in the report by Giggs (1973: 1210-12) of a study of schizophrenia among immigrants in Nottingham. In this study he used hospital-based admissions to examine the difference between the rates of schizophrenia in native-born whites and other ethnic groups. This, however, makes the assumption that all schizophrenics would in fact receive hospital care. This may not be true, simply because for the period chosen not all schizophrenics were identified, purely because the severity of their illness was not sufficient to require admission.

With changes in practice in the care of psychiatric illness, patients have gradually moved from custodial to community care, with the hospital playing a role more in the acute episode than in long-term care. Thus, more community care is now practised between general practitioners and community-based psychiatric clinics. This has led, in some places, to the establishment of case registers which have become a source for collecting morbidity data, but it will be quickly recognised that the number of people on the case register will be related to the availability of the community-based services. Thus, in the enumeration of cases there may be limitations as to the accuracy of the case registers in reflecting the prevalence or incidence of a particular disease.

Identification of Unknown Cases.   In essence this involves the same principles of screening which will be outlined in Chapter 8 and case definition is a fundamental part of this particular exercise. Cooper and Morgan (1973: 38) suggest that there is an under-reporting of mental illness due to a failure to recognise cases and also the problem of deciding when the state of abnormality is reached. The methods involved in screening a population for illness are outlined in detail in Chapter 8 and the identification of psychiatric illness by these methods does, in itself, have limitations, particularly in relation to the definition of a case.

The problems of epidemiological studies in respect of psychiatric illness are considerable, principally because of the multifactorial nature of the problem, which makes case definition difficult. Attempts have been made to overcome these problems and studies have been used to help in the assessment of the amount of psychiatric illness in a population and hence the planning of psychiatric services. Epidemiological studies may give some estimate of the likely workload from certain common psychiatric illnesses arising within a population, and in the next section some of the studies which have been undertaken will be discussed briefly.

Epidemiological Studies and Planning of Services

In the previous section attention was drawn to the work of Frerichs *et al* (1981) in Los Angeles, where they found different prevalence rates for depression amongst different ethnic and socio-economic groups. The relevance of this type of information for health care planners must be seen not wholly in the context of more hospital beds, but in the totality of provision of care by both medical and social workers. In addition, the identification that environmental factors may be concerned indicates that local authorities should be involved in a much broader context, for example in housing policies.

Dean and James (1980: 167-80) studied the distribution of depressive illness in the City of Plymouth. In this study they were able to plot on maps the areas of the city where depressive illness was high and low, and to correlate these with social, economic, age and sex factors. For example, the incidence of depression was found to be higher in women than in men. In men depression tended to occur amongst the more elderly age groups, who were also socially isolated (living alone) and of low socio-economic status. In women, the illness occurred mostly in unmarried women in the low socio-economic grouping, where family stress was thought to be a factor. Clearly such studies as this and those in Los

Angeles produce vital information, not only for examining services in terms of provision, but also the cause of the illness itself. Nielsen and Nielsen (1977: 491-503) carried out a detailed study of the use of psychiatric services and mental illness on the island of Samsø in Denmark. Their findings also indicated higher prevalence of mental illness, based on hospital data, amongst lower socio-economic groups. They found that approximately 12.7 per cent of the population had been referred to the psychiatric services and that schizophrenia was diagnosed in two per thousand of the population and psychoses of all types in 30 per thousand.

Watts (1966: 30-3) undertook a study of depressive disorders in a general practice in Leicestershire and estimated that psychiatric illness accounted for 7-10 per cent of all practice contacts, but indicated that this was for a predominantly rural practice. Of this proportion, about 25 per cent was due to depressive illness and Watts suggested that this illness had a prevalence rate of approximately 12 per thousand in his practice. Studies of depressive illness have shown a variation in respect of the proportion of people involved (prevalence rate), though there has been a consistency in terms of the factors associated with depressive illness and the distribution of the illness in the population. McMullen (1976: 504-8) in a study in Aberdeen, found that social classes IV and V were more likely to suffer from evidence of depression than were the higher social classes. This finding is similar to that by Nielsen *et al* (1977), Dean *et al* (1980) and Frerichs *et al* (1981). In addition, he also found, as had the other studies, that women were more likely to suffer from depressive illness than men, and that the range was between 1.8:1 and 2:1. Women were more likely to be in the younger age group than men and socio-economic factors were important in the distribution of depressive illness, as indicated above.

These studies give some indication of the likely workload arising in a population from this particular illness, and show that there are variations in terms of the likely prevalence depending on whether the practice is rural or urban and if there are any particular problems in the urban situation. To this extent the information may give an indicator to planners as to whether more community-based psychiatric clinics and additional community psychiatric nurses would benefit the service provision and help prevent this illness, or whether joint care planning activity is needed between local authority and health services to provide better housing and more support from social workers.

Community studies have been important in planning services for psychiatric illness and for the mentally handicapped, and an example has been the work of Kushlick (1966: 73-82) in respect of services for the mentally subnormal in the Wessex region. His studies found that there were 17 per 100,000 severely subnormal patients aged 0-15 years living in hostel or hospital accommodation, and suggested that some of these patients might be cared for other than in the traditional hospital setting, and recommended small social units. Kushlick also found that the prevalence of severe subnormality had gradually decreased over the years, despite an increase in the prevalence of Down's syndrome. These changes in the prevalence suggested the interaction of different factors. One possibility for the fall in the overall prevalence rate might have been related to advances in obstetric care. The increase in the prevalence of Down's syndrome could be due to the availability of antibiotics to treat chest diseases, to which mongols are prone, and to which, prior to antibiotics, they often succumbed. Thus, increased survival was the main factor. This type of detailed study into one particular aspect of psychiatric illness was to lead to the development, in Wessex, of small social units for the care of the severely mentally handicapped, assessing suitable patients from the hospital population. This policy has led to the gradual reduction in the number of hospital places that are required for this group of psychiatrically ill patients. In addition, the work has had benefit in producing a register of severely mentally handicapped people, such that health and social services are able to discuss programmes of activity in terms of providing a more comprehensive service for this particular group.

The Role of Nurses in the Community.   Clarke (1980: 98-100) discussed the role of health visitors and the need for the group to become involved in the management and recognition of psychiatric illness within the population they were responsible for. Health visitors have, within their training programme, a requirement to understand the prevention of mental, physical and emotional ill-health or the alleviation of its consequences, and this must imply that they understand the aetiology of the illnesses with which they will be concerned and their distribution within the population as a whole. Thus, it is important for them to recognise that depression is more likely to be found in young women and in older men, and that socio-economic and ethnic culture may also play a part in the aetiology and distribution of the disease.

Some workers suggested that an indication of the failure to identify depressive illness was the number of suicides which occurred in England and Wales. Table 7.9 analyses mortality from suicides and self-inflicted injuries per million of the population between 1952 and 1975. The figures indicate that the rate of suicide has in fact been falling. Does this suggest that:

(1) There is better recognition at an early stage of depressive illness, and hence treatment preventing suicide, or

(2) Is it that there is better treatment for those who attempt suicide and death is prevented by medical care, or

(3) Could this be that there has in fact been a continual decline in the incidence of suicides for other reasons such as improvement in social conditions?

Table 7.9: England and Wales: Deaths from Suicide and Self-Inflicted Injuries per Million of the Population for Selected Years 1952 to 1975.

Suicides and Self-Inflicted Injuries	1952	1955	1962	1965	1972	1975
Number	4338	5000	5588	5261	3770	3693
Rate	99	113	120	110	77	75

Sources: (a) Registrar General's Report, *Tables Medical 1952, 1955, 1962, 1965, 1972*, HMSO, London. (b) Office of Population Censuses and Surveys, *Mortality Statistics: Cause 1975*, Table 2.

These are some of the aspects of psychiatric illness where community nurses can play an important part in the collection of information about psychiatric illness within their community practice. As Clarke (1980) suggested recognition of psychiatric illness is highly important and that is dependent upon an understanding of the epidemiology of psychiatric illness. Basically, therefore, the basic questions: who?, when?, where? and why? can be applied to psychiatric illness to determine the distribution and attempt to provide answers to the question of the cause, but as has been indicated, there are certain special problems in the study of psychiatric illness.

8 SCREENING FOR DISEASE IN A COMMUNITY

The Concept of Screening

The term screening (as applied to the investigation of disease) can be defined as: the application of one or more, usually simple and standard, investigations to generally large numbers of individuals who do not have specific symptoms of disease, but who attend in the hope of obtaining benefit. The investigations are designed to reveal people who have the disease but may not have any symptoms (asymptomatic) from within the population who attend.

For any particular disease occurring in a population those with the disease can be grouped into three categories: those known to the general practitioner services; those known to the hospital services (which includes some known to the general practitioner services); and those not known to either health care agency. The distribution of these three groups can be represented diagrammatically as in Figure 8.1.

Figure 8.1: Distribution of Disease in a Population

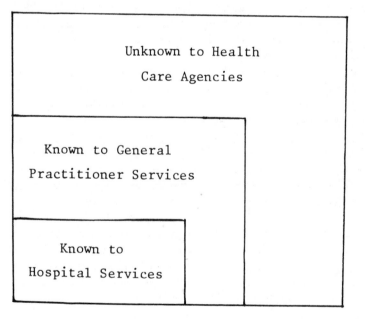

Unknown to Health
Care Agencies

Known to General
Practitioner Services

Known to
Hospital Services

The distribution within these groups will vary according to the severity of the disease in the individuals affected and their perception of illness (ill-health as related to symptoms).

Coronary heart disease presenting as acute myocardial infarction (heart attack) will be substantially represented in the 'hospital and general practitioner' group, with only a small proportion in the 'unknown to health care agency' group. Conversely people suffering from the 'common cold' will be substantially represented (unless there are complications) in the 'unknown to health care agency' group, because they do not seek medical care. To some extent, therefore, the presentation of disease to one of the health care agencies may depend not only on the recognition of disease by the individual but the known effectiveness of treatment.

Within the population in the 'unknown to health care agencies' group there will be a range of severity of symptoms amongst the individuals suffering from the disease under study. This severity will range from: those whose symptoms are of sufficient severity to make them actively consider seeking care, those with minimal symptoms which are noticed but considered bearable and those who have not yet noticed symptoms but have the disease. This last group do not seek medical care because they have no symptoms and are in the 'asymptomatic phase' of the disease whilst the other two groups do have symptoms which they notice.

Screening programmes try specifically to identify the group who have the disease but no symptoms. Thus screening in identifying this group of people aims to allow the disease to be arrested through treatment or removal of a risk factor before irreversible changes have occurred. To this extent screening is a 'secondary preventive measure', in that people who already have the disease or are at risk to the disease, compared to others in the population, are identified and treatment given to alter the natural course of the disease.

Screening does not, however, in all cases fulfil this concept of arresting the progress of disease. The programme may identify individuals in whom the disease is irreversible and treatment not effective, but benefits can be offered, for example screening for deafness in children. Thus, screening may be considered under the following groupings:

Screening for Individuals with Disease needing Treatment. Screening in this instance identifies those people who have a disease which is asymptomatic but requires active treatment to prevent it progressing. The disease is established and could affect not only the individual but also the community, for example tuberculosis.

Screening for Individuals Developing the Disease.   Screening in this context identifies individuals who are developing the disease, have early changes in the normal physiological processes which could, unchecked, lead to irreversible change. For example, early screening for raised blood pressure, which could be a precursor to the development of hypertensive heart disease and stroke.

Screening for Individuals with Irreversible Disease but who may Benefit from Care.   In this context the process of screening tries to identify people with irreversible disease for which care may be offered which improves their social functioning. For example, the screening for deafness in children identifies a group of individuals for whom educational and technical help are available which can improve their social and educational attainments, particularly if care can be started early.

Screening for At-risk Groups.   Screening in this context tries to identify those people who may exhibit or personally practise habits which are known to be detrimental to health, for example obesity and cigarette smoking. The screening of these at-risk groups within a population may allow education and persuasion to be used to influence the individuals to change their habits and reduce the risk of developing the disease. At this stage the individual may have no symptoms but the risk of developing symptoms is greater than in individuals abstaining from the habit.

Thus, screening may apparently not (under these headings) be as simplistic a concept as the definition used at the beginning. However, the definition does stand the test in as much as each of the four sub-headings requires identification of an individual by some investigation, and the individual can benefit from care of some sort. Thus, screening differs from most other clinical forms of care in that the purpose of the investigation is to diagnose the disease early by simple investigations which in themselves are *not* a form of treatment. The arrest of progress is dependent upon treatment being available of one form or another.

Screening also differs from other forms of care in that it is not sought by the public, but is offered to the public in an attempt to reduce the affect of a particular disease in the population. If an individual accepts the invitation to the programme, then he/she expects to receive benefit. This concept raises a number of issues related to the establishment of a screening programme, the disease and treatment.

Screening – Issues to be Considered in Relation to the Disease under Investigation

The identification of the disease in its asymptomatic state through a screening investigation has as an objective the possibility of offering treatment or care and altering the natural course of the disease. This presupposes, however, that a number of important aspects are known about the disease itself. These are considered in the following paragraphs.

What is a Case?

Screening tries to identify those people with a disease and in the rest of this chapter this will relate to those whose disease is in the early stage of development. The purpose of screening in these cases is to prevent the disease from progressing by early treatment. As indicated earlier, disease exists in all grades of severity so that at some stage a decision has to be made to define the changes which warrant intervention – that is the state changes from normal to abnormal and that abnormal state can be termed a 'case'.

The definition of a case of a particular disease needs a clinical description of the abnormal state. This may be based upon clinical signs and/or abnormality of some physiological measurement, indicating that the individual has passed from a normal to an abnormal physiological state. In respect of a screening programme aimed at identifying people with early signs of high blood pressure (hypertension), the point at which the diastolic blood pressure changes from normal to abnormal would need to be defined, if this was the sole measurement to be used in the screening programme.

The measurement may not be a physical one; however, in the screening programme for cervical cancer, measurement is made of cell structure. Again, a defined change or changes in the composition of cervical cells obtained from a cervical smear are looked for as indicators of change from normal to abnormal. Whatever measurement is used the principle is to identify the stage which is defined as the change from a normal to an abnormal state.

What is the Natural Course of the Disease?

An essential factor in the consideration of establishing a screening programme for a particular disease is knowledge of what is the natural course (history) of that disease. If a disease appears, produces symptoms and then regresses and disappears leaving no residual disability, then the need for a screening programme may not be justified. Thus, an investigator would wish to know whether the disease spontaneously regresses if left untreated, progresses rapidly (acute) or slowly (chronic). Without an understanding of the natural course of the disease a decision cannot be made as to whether a screening programme, with associated early treatment, would be beneficial. For example, some types of leukaemias are of sudden acute onset, and progress rapidly to a fatal outcome. At present it is unlikely that routine screening programmes would be effective in identifying the disease in early stages, as more knowledge may be required of the course from the normal to abnormal state.

This problem of the length of the asymptomatic phase of the disease raises the issue of how often and who should be screened to determine if changes are taking place. At present the intervals between screenings for cervical cancer in women over 35 years of age is three years, whilst for men who work in the rubber industry and are at risk of bladder cancer, screening of urine is recommended every six months.

Diseases with acute onset are less likely to be suitable for screening programmes as the asymptomatic phase will be short. Exceptions to this rule are the inherited diseases appearing in early infancy, for example phenylketonuria. In this condition it is essential to identify children with the disease as early in life as possible, to prevent irreversible changes in mental ability. Early detection can lead to early treatment and prevention of the natural course.

Does Early Treatment Improve Prognosis?

Some diseases are known to occur more frequently in certain groups of the population, for example bladder cancer amongst people who have worked in the rubber industry. These groups can be considered to be 'at risk' of developing the disease. Consideration must be given, however, to the question as to whether early treatment will bring benefit. For example, techniques are available to screen within a population for those individuals who are likely to develop diabetes mellitus, therefore identifying people with asymptomatic disease. If early treatment is given to this group do they benefit from the treatment and is their risk of premature death from complicating factors reduced, when compared to the normal population or to those individuals presenting as an acute case? If the answer is 'no' then the justification for screening becomes less.

For each particular disease-screening programme there needs to be an investigation as to whether the early detection and subsequent treatment carry any benefit to the individual, when set against the known natural course of the disease. A screening programme which can recognise asymptomatic disease may not be justified if the early treatment affords no benefit, as the prognosis is not altered.

Is the Screening Programme Justifiable?

Some of these aspects have been raised under the previous headings, but there are some additional factors which need consideration.

Can the National Health Service afford the Programme? This aspect can be considered not only in purely financial terms of the capital and revenue costs of establishing and running the programme, but also whether the population benefit from its establishment, when compared to some other proposed service development. An example of the complexity of the issues can be illustrated by the screening programme for phenylketonuria in infants. When unidentified in infants, this disease progresses and causes the children to become mentally retarded. This outcome then requires provision of special facilities for caring for this group, not only within the Health Service but also local authority. However, treatment is available, if the disease is detected early, which is not expensive and allows normal development of the affected children. The screening investigation is cheap to administer and process. Thus, in introducing the programme the cost had to be balanced against the long-term costs of non-treatment. In each situation these types of conflicts have to be decided and the advantages and disadvantages weighed up within the overall financial constraints within the National Health Service.

Are Facilities available for Treatment? Screening programmes in themselves are not a form of treatment, they are diagnostic procedures. Thus, in considering the introduction of a screening programme not only has the question of the type of treatment available to be considered, but the facilities within which to carry out that treatment if it is necessary. An example of this would be in relation to screening for breast cancer. If the assumption is made that the screening programme would identify people with 'lumps' in the breast, then to confirm the diagnosis this would require biopsy and histological studies of the tissue removed. Clearly this requires in-patient and pathology facilities and has implications, therefore, on a number of departments and on the admission of other patients with other conditions. Ethically there is, therefore, a requirement to ensure that if treatment is available, facilities to carry out that treatment should be available.

Who should be included in the programme?   In considering a screening programme account must be taken of the group(s) within the population who are to be included in the screening programme. This may be the total population, as in the case of newborn babies being screened for phenylketonuria or hypothyroidism. Conversely it may be special groups such as people who work in the rubber industry, at risk to bladder cancer.

Evidence suggests that for some programmes the original groups included might have been too limited, as in the case of cervical cancer, where initially it was limited to women over 35 years of age. Recent evidence from the Office of Population Censuses and Surveys (1982: 2) relating to the incidence of various types of cancer suggests that the incidence of cervical cancer has been increasing in the age group 25-34 years, an age group not previously covered by screening. New evidence has now shown that in fact women under the age of 35 years are being screened the most intensively (Roberts 1982: 41-3), indicating that some screening programmes need to be constantly reviewed in the light of new epidemiological information.

Investigations Used in Screening

A major consideration in the development of a screening programme is the type of investigation to be used. There are a number of factors to be considered in relation to the investigation, for example cost, acceptability and validity. These will be discussed in this section.

Types of Investigations

The following investigations have been used in screening programmes and are presented as examples. Their use in a particular screening programme would need to be assessed against the criteria for an investigation (which are discussed). Where possible alternative investigations should be available (reference investigation) to allow the accuracy of the screening investigation to be checked.

Questionnaires.   These are printed forms containing specific questions to try and identify whether an individual may be suffering from the disease under study. These may be either completed by an interviewer in direct contact with individuals, or sent through the post (postal questionnaire) asking individuals to complete the forms and return them.

Physical Examinations.   These are investigations applied directly to an individual, for example blood pressure measurement, hearing and vision assessments, lung function tests.

Laboratory Investigations.   These investigations rely on an individual providing a sample of tissue or body fluid for laboratory investigation. This may involve detailed procedures and may involve 'invasive techniques', for example venepuncture. Examples of laboratory investigations include urinalysis, blood analysis, cytological examinations of tissues.

X-ray Investigations.   These are complex investigations requiring sophisticated resources. They have been used, particularly in the past, to screen from populations those individuals suffering from tuberculosis. Today other techniques have been developed, for example thermography and ultrasound, which do not use X-rays and hence reduce any risk from the exposure to X-rays.

Anthropomorphic Investigations.   These are measurements related to body size or parts of the body, for example head circumference, body-fat thickness, height and weight.

The different types of measurement may be used alone or in multiples (multiphasic screening). When considering their use, they need to be assessed against certain criteria, which they should fulfil.

Criteria for Assessing an Investigation

The criteria against which an investigation needs to be assessed are important to ensure that the investigation used in the programme does what it was designed to do and does it effectively. The criteria against which the investigation should be assessed are discussed.

Simplicity.   The investigation should be as simple as possible to administer, whether it is a questionnaire or a physical examination. Complex investigations are often unacceptable because of cost, administration and time necessary to carry them out.

Accuracy.   The investigation used should be as reasonably true a measurement of the attribute as possible.

Repeatability.   The investigation should be repeatable and produce the same results accurately over a long period of time.

Acceptability.   The investigation should be such that it will be acceptable to the population who are being screened. Acceptability of an
investigation helps to obtain a satisfactory response from the population to the screening programme. A complex test may be unacceptable
and provoke anxiety and hence a low response rate.

Validity.   The investigation and the results it produces need to be monitored and checked by a reference investigation.

Cost.   The investigation should, in financial terms, be as cheap to administer as possible.

Yield.   The ideal investigation should identify those people at risk
(with asymptomatic disease) without having to examine large numbers
of people. Sometimes this is not possible if the disease has a low prevalence in the population, but the seriousness of the condition may
justify such an operation. Phenylketonuria has an incidence of about
1 in 10,000 live births, but because of its potentially damaging effect if
undetected it is justifiable to screen for this disease. Conversely Wilson's
disease, with a prevalence of 1:100,000 in children, is too low a prevalence to warrant mass screening (Balke and Howell-Wright 1963; Raine
1975).

Does the Investigation reach the Group(s) at Risk?   The investigation
should reach those groups at risk. For example cancer of the cervix is
known to be related to social class, particularly groups IV and V. Evidence by Wigfield (1976: 65-73) suggests that the screening programme
may not be effective amongst this group, that is the groups at risk are
not receiving the investigation.

   These criteria should act as guidelines when assessing the suitability
of an investigation for a programme. Equally, however, the investigation
and the programme need to be evaluated.

Evaluation of a Screening Programme

The basic tool of the screening programme is the investigation(s) employed to identify individuals with the disease under study. In discussing the criteria for an investigation in a screening programme, attention
was drawn to the need for accuracy, repeatability and validity as well as
the need for a reference investigation for comparison of the results. The
reference investigation allows this comparison to be made using two
measures: specificity and sensitivity.

Specificity. The specificity of an investigation may be defined as the proportion of true negative (healthy) individuals correctly identified. A specific test should, therefore, yield few false positives when it is used, otherwise there will be a high over-referral rate for further investigations, which may cause unnecessary anxiety to individuals.

Sensitivity. The sensitivity of an investigation may be defined as the proportion of true positive (diseased) individuals correctly identified. A sensitive test should, therefore, yield few false negatives. Ideally a test should be highly sensitive and highly specific. In practice there is compromise.

The relationship between sensitivity and specificity is illustrated diagrammatically in Table 8.1. The table illustrates the way in which the two measures are calculated, using a tabular form comparing the screening investigation against the reference investigation. As indicated earlier, the reference investigation may be another laboratory investigation or a full clinical examination. In practice a balance is aimed for between the specificity and sensitivity of an investigation.

Table 8.1: Specificity and Sensitivity of a Screening Investigation

		Results of the reference test	
		Disease present (+ve)	Disease absent (−ve)
Results of Screening Test	Disease present (+ve)	True positives (a)	False positives (b)
	Disease absent (−ve)	False negatives (c)	True negatives (d)

Note: Sensitivity — Proportion correctly identified as positive = $\frac{a}{a+c}$ × 100

Specificity — Proportion correctly identified as negative = $\frac{d}{b+d}$ × 100

Over-referral rate or false positive rate = $\frac{b}{a+b}$ × 100

Under-referral rate or false negative rate = $\frac{c}{c+d}$ × 100

In some instances improvement in the sensitivity will reduce the specificity and lead to an increase in false positives — people being referred unnecessarily for further examination. If the investigation is cheap in financial terms, acceptable and simple to carry out, a high sensitivity may be acceptable, providing the reference investigation is readily available and easy to perform, to distinguish the true from the false positives. In a screening trial for breast cancer using palpation alone as the investigation, a 67 per cent sensitivity rate was achieved. If palpation was combined with mammography the sensitivity rate was raised, but this was at the expense of a high false positive rate (over-referral rate), which approached 76 per cent (Roberts 1977: 86-9).

The relative values of the specificity and sensitivity of a test will need to be determined, based on both statistical and medical advice and the values (ranges) acceptable as being within normal and abnormal limits. This relationship between the specificity and sensitivity is termed the 'predictive value'. The predictive value is dependent upon the prevalence of the disease being studied.

A low prevalence of a disease in the population may give rise to an unexpectedly high false positive rate (over-referrals), so the specificity value might not be the appropriate value. By altering the range of the limits between what is accepted as normal or abnormal, the over-referral rate might be reduced, but the numbers might remain too high. This may have to be accepted, however, if a 100 per cent sensitivity is set for the investigation where the disease occurs only once in 1,000 or 10,000 times. Such values may give an over-referral rate of 25 to 1, but the reduction in sensitivity may not be acceptable. The correct balance is acquired by consultation with a statistician, bearing in mind that the clinical importance may outweigh statistical perfection.

The Nurse's Role in Screening

Nurses and health visitors have a particularly important role to play in screening programmes, particularly in respect of education and the administration of the investigations.

Education

Nurses need to know the context in which screening programmes have been established, the investigations that are used, the benefits to those individuals identified as being abnormal and the treatment available. This background knowledge is essential if nurses are to carry out an educative role within the population and to particular groups at risk. In this capacity they are also practising preventive medicine, even though at a secondary level. Conversely a nurse needs to know why screening programmes may *not* have been introduced, for example cost, accuracy, low prevalence of the disease in the population or inability to provide proven benefit by early treatment.

Practical Application

Nurses are often actively involved in the application of screening tests to individuals in the population. This requires special training and under-standing of the techniques and the reasons for being precise about the way the investigation is carried out. In addition there is a need for nurses and other health care professionals to appreciate that, while an individual is undergoing the investigation, reassurance and a high standard of professional discipline are essential. Inadvertent remarks may cause quite unintentional anxiety to the individual. The nurse, through her skills in inter-personal relationships, can have a marked effect on the level of uptake of a screening programme and is an essen-tial member of a team. This is particularly true in respect of community-based nurses (health visitors and district nurses).

Screening is the principal method of secondary prevention — that is the prevention of disease already evident in a person from progressing to gross pathological change. As indicated previously, this requires a detailed knowledge of the natural course of the disease and what treat-ment is available. Screening is not a simple procedure and the diseases for which screening programmes have been suggested are indicated in Table 8.2. Pressure to introduce further screening programmes may become even greater as the population begins to age, but these pro-grammes need to be rigidly assessed against the criteria outlined and knowledge of the disease.

Table 8.2: *England and Wales: Some Examples of Diseases where Screen-ing Investigations are Currently Used*

Phenylketonuria in infants
Hypothyroidism in infants
Hearing in infants
Vision in infants
Congenital dislocation of the hip
Cervical cancer in women
Bladder cancer in males who have worked in the rubber industry

9 PREVENTION OF DISEASE IN A COMMUNITY

What is Prevention?

Prevention of disease may be considered as a number of mechanisms by which ill-health is prevented from occurring or progressing in an individual or population. This implies there is some understanding of the cause of the event though this understanding may often be incomplete. When the concept of prevention is applied to disease in a community, then the role of the epidemiologist becomes extremely important, since the principle of the epidemiologist's practice is the study of the distribution and determinants of disease in man. A basic view might be taken that once the cause of a disease is known, then it can usually be prevented, though the means to effect this could be long-term.

Evidence has shown that for many diseases, the discovery of the cause has led to their control or even eradication from within populations. Control does not, however, imply eradication but, as will be considered, is associated with the concepts of the prevention of disease. The most recent and exciting example of disease control and eradication has been in respect of smallpox. At the 33rd World Health Assembly of the World Health Organisation in May 1980 it was announced that, following an independent scientific investigation, smallpox had been finally eradicated worldwide, through a long-term policy of population vaccination (Breman and Arita 1980: 1263-73). This process of eradication of smallpox had taken over 200 years to achieve on a worldwide basis. For other diseases, for example cancers, skin diseases and accidents, the picture is different. Knowledge of the cause in many instances still remains inadequately understood, and whilst medical care can be used to treat an individual and perhaps cure or relieve the symptoms, prevention of the disease actually occurring in the individual or the community as a whole has not yet been achieved. Thus, in the discussion of the prevention of disease within a community it is possible to consider this in terms of infectious and non-infectious diseases.

A more detailed examination of the concept of prevention suggests the spectrum of control of the disease within communities which may at one end involve actual elimination of the disease and at the other the provision of medical care to treat individuals with the disease, controlling that disease and preventing its normal course of progress (natural

104

history). This in itself suggests that there may be different levels for the prevention of disease in a community, with different emphases on the methods of prevention as well as considering the different aetiological factors (infectious or non-infectious).

For some diseases, for example accidents, a three-tier level of prevention could be envisaged. The first level would be to prevent the accident happening, the second level to reduce the possibility of injury or death if an accident did occur and the third to provide medical care, in the event of injury occurring in an accident, to try and restore normal function. This concept is summarised in Figure 9.1. In this chapter, however, the problems of prevention and its levels will focus on acute infectious and non-infectious diseases and exclude accidents, since this group of diseases is not entirely characteristic in terms of the levels of prevention compared to the other acute diseases.

Figure 9.1: Levels of Prevention Related to Accidents

LEVEL 1   Primary Prevention — To prevent the accident occurring
           (Education, Engineering, Legislation)

LEVEL 2   Secondary Prevention — To prevent or reduce injury in the event of
           an accident occurring
           (Seat belts, Crash Helmets, Bust-proof Locks)

LEVEL 3   Tertiary Prevention — To prevent serious pathological consequences
           resulting from the injuries sustained
           (Treatment)

Levels of Prevention of Disease in a Community

Figure 9.1 has suggested that there are various levels at which the preventive activity may take place. These include the community level whereby, through education, engineering and legislation, the community is made aware of the factors associated with the disease (accidents) and hence the hope is that the disease will be prevented from occurring. This concept remains true in respect of acute diseases and is equivalent to the primary prevention level in Figure 9.1. Obviously this involves the co-operation of individuals in the prevention of disease, thus reducing the community's risk to that disease.

Figure 9.1 also indicated a second level which suggested the reduction in the effect on the individual if exposed to and contracting the disease. This level is intermediary between primary prevention and what in this chapter will be termed secondary prevention, namely the treatment of the individual with the disease, which is shown as level three in Figure 9.1.

Thus, in respect of acute diseases other than accidents, two levels of prevention will be considered. These are: primary prevention, concerned with protecting individuals within communities and hence the community as a whole from actually contracting the disease; and secondary prevention, which is concerned with the organisation of treatment services for an individual who has contracted the disease. Thus, in this latter group prevention is concerned with diminishing, if possible, the pathological consequences of the disease and restoring the individual to a state of normal health.

Chapter 2 has outlined how the prevention of some diseases has altered the pattern of mortality and morbidity in this country, with a decline in mortality from infectious diseases, but a rise in mortality from non-infectious ones. The elimination or control of cholera, diphtheria, enteric fever (typhoid and paratyphoid), scarlet fever and tuberculosis, are examples of the control and prevention of infectious-type diseases. The control of non-infectious diseases is, however, more complex and amongst these can be considered the occupational diseases and social diseases such as smoking and alcoholism. In the publication by the Department of Health and Social Security, *Prevention and Health, Everybody's Business* (1976), the requirement still to maintain vigilance in controlling infectious disease is highlighted, as well as the problem of controlling the non-infectious diseases now affecting our society. The concepts of primary and secondary prevention, as outlined above, will be discussed separately, indicating how the two are interlinked.

Primary Prevention

Primary prevention tries, through knowledge of the cause of the disease, to eradicate that disease from the community or to provide protection to the individuals forming that community, protecting them from being affected by the disease and thereby giving rise to clinical symptoms and ill-health. The methods for achieving this end may include 'immunisation' — protecting the individual, which may lead to eradication of the disease in man; 'eradication' — by population immunisation and other methods; and 'quarantine' — the isolation of people who have been in contact with the disease from the rest of the community. The two main methods of prevention used today are eradication and immunisation, though quarantine still has an important, though smaller role, to play than in previous times.

Eradication. This method of prevention aims to remove the disease completely from within the community. The processes involved may be complex and require clear knowledge and understanding of the cause of the disease, including the life-cycle and natural history of the organism(s) causing the disease. Mention has been made of the world-wide eradication of smallpox in man, which was achieved by mass immunisation to render the population immune to the virus causing smallpox. The natural history of the disease showed that man was the host for the organism so that by rendering him immune the organism was no longer able to infect him and thus continue to be transmitted.

Eradication may, however, be limited purely to groups of individuals, for example those working in a particular occupation. The discovery of the association between the use of a chemical substance and a specific disease has led to the banning and removal of that substance, either voluntarily or through legislation, and thus in the longer term to the eradication of that disease in that group of workers. The use of the compound naphthylamine in the rubber industry was found to be associated with bladder cancer and this compound was subsequently withdrawn from use (Lock and Smith 1977: 159). A further example of the way in which disease prevention and possible eradication in industry has been carried out, has been the recognition of the association between asbestos and lung cancer. Legislation has been introduced to control the use of this substance and codes of industrial hygiene have been recommended in respect of the processing of asbestos for industrial and other uses (Newhouse 1979: 59-70).

Eradication may also involve an indirect attack on the life-cycle of the organism causing the disease as, for example, in the case of malaria. Whilst drugs may be given prophylactically to visitors of areas of endemic malaria, a great deal of attention has been paid to the eradication of the mosquito which is known to be in the chain of transmission. Though man, once infected, acts as a reservoir, transmission between man and man is through the mosquito, which carries infected blood and infects other people when it bites them in search of its blood meal (Parry 1973: 156-9).

In England and Wales the eradication of water-borne diseases, such as typhoid, cholera and dysentery, has principally been due to engineering combined with the chemical treatment of water, to provide 'pure' water. Whilst sporadic outbreaks of typhoid do still occur, these are generally due to people who are carriers of the disease transmitting the disease to other people, or to people returning from endemic areas who are incubating the disease (Haward and Schofield 1978: 181-5).

Eradication is one of the principal aims of primary prevention and for some diseases this can be achieved directly by immunisation or indirectly through attacking part of the life-cycle of the organism, as has been attempted with malaria. Eradication may require education, legislation and engineering processes, singly or together. Education remains one of the primary methods of trying to effect eradication, whether it is the control of the disease leading to its eventual eradication in a whole population, for example smallpox in India (Basu, Jezek and Ward 1979: 187-233) or the problem of cross-infection in an operating theatre. If eradication cannot be achieved simply then immunisation may be required in conjunction with other measures. This process, however, is principally concerned with infectious disease.

Immunisation.   This is a primary preventive measure of particular importance in the prevention of infectious disease, because the process of inducing immunity to the disease protects people from contracting that disease and having clinical symptoms. In some diseases the immunity that can be given does not totally prevent clinical symptoms but alters the natural course of the disease, reducing the severity of the clinical symptoms, for example in measles.

The use of a vaccine in immunising children against measles has been shown to modify the attack of measles, but subsequently in an outbreak of measles some children, even though vaccinated, may still show clinical symptoms of measles, though generally less severe than the unvaccinated population. The possible reasons for this occurrence are speculate but the improper storage of a vaccine can reduce its potency and hence the protection it would give, the organism may change its virulence – the vaccine being less effective, and the children may have a defective immune mechanism which does not produce an adequate number of antibodies to overcome the infection when it presents.

An additional factor is that even when a person is immunised and antibodies are produced, over a period of time, if that person is not in contact with the disease or reimmunised, the antibody levels gradually fall off and the body does not react when challenged by the organism. Thus, the use of immunisation as a primary preventive measure requires a knowledge of the immunological response that is likely to occur within an individual and for how long that response – the production of antibodies – will last. (The acquisition of immunity will be discussed later in this chapter.)

Quarantine.   The principle of this method is to isolate from the community those who are known, or are suspected, of having been in contact with people suffering from the disease. This principle of prevention is specifically related to the control of infectious disease and quarantine and isolation of people with infectious disease has been practised for many centuries. Evidence from medieval times indicates that persons suffering from leprosy (lepers) were isolated from the community and were in fact considered to be legally dead (Singer 1928: 78-80). With the growth in trading in the eighteenth and nineteenth centuries quarantine of ships before they could enter ports became a regular practice, particularly if they had come from areas of the world where infectious disease, such as smallpox, cholera, were endemic.

Quarantine, therefore, involves the isolation of those suspected of having been in contact with an infectious disease and hence may be developing the disease (incubating). This requires them to be quarantined until the period of incubation is passed and indicates whether they have developed the disease or not. International concern over the spread of infectious disease, particularly in the late nineteenth and early twentieth centuries, led in 1907 to the formation in Paris of the Office International d'Hygiene Publique to provide information on an international basis about infectious diseases. This office was, in 1948, absorbed into the World Health Organisation, which still maintains a worldwide role of monitoring infectious disease (Cartwright 1977: 186-7).

Secondary Prevention

At this level prevention is concerned with trying to prevent the pathological consequences of the disease which has afflicted the individual. This requires a knowledge of the natural course of the disease (natural history) in order to try and provide an effective treatment, intervening in the natural course of the disease. For some diseases it is possible to directly intervene and eradicate the disease, for example the treatment of tuberculosis with drugs. In other infectious diseases of viral origin there is currently no effective cure and the natural course of the disease occurs. One benefit may be that the individual will gain immunity to further attacks (acquired immunity), for example in mumps and measles. In other cases, for example influenza or the common cold, no such long-lasting immunity occurs. Secondary prevention, therefore, in the context of acute infectious disease, is primarily concerned with the treatment or management of the clinical manifestations and where possible the alteration of the natural course of the disease to eradicate it from an individual. As indicated previously, however, for many infectious diseases, particularly of viral origin, eradication is not possible and

in these circumstances treatment may only slow down the natural pro-
gression of the disease.

One result of contact with a disease and the occurrence of clinical
symptoms is that acquired immunity may result. Immunisation (the
obtaining of immunity) and eradication are the two major weapons
in terms of the control of infectious disease, and the immunity of an
individual or a community to disease is an essential factor in primary
prevention. The acquisition of immunity, therefore, is important and
this is outlined below.

Infectious Disease and Immunity

Immunity may be considered as a form of resistance which an individual
may have to a specific micro-organism, which depends upon the presence in the individual of antibodies which have an exclusive inactivating
action on that specific micro-organism or its products (toxins). The
micro-organism or its products are termed the antigen and they provoke
the body's defence mechanism to produce antibodies which in effect
inactivate the antigen and prevent the pathological changes and development of clinical symptoms (normally associated with that micro-
organism or its products). The study of the antigen-antibody response
is called immunology. Various laboratory techniques are available, for
example agglutination, complement fixation and precipitation tests. The
immunologist can then establish whether antibodies to specific antigens
are present in an individual's blood and hence assess their immune state.

The immunity of an individual to a specific disease may arise in a
variety of ways; immunity may be inherited or may be acquired naturally or artificially. These different ways of obtaining immunity and
their relevance to prevention of the disease will be discussed briefly and
Table 9.1 summarises how immunity can occur.

Table 9.1: Summary of Methods by which Immunity may be Acquired

(1) Inherited:	Genetic make-up determines susceptibility to disease(s)
(2) Naturally acquired:	(a) From direct infection by the micro-organism (active)
	(b) From mother during development of foetus (passive) and from breast milk
(3) Artificially acquired:	(a) Immunisation — antibodies injected to give immed- iate protection, but not long-lasting (passive)
	(b) Immunisation — live or killed micro-organisms or their products injected to provoke antibody response (active)

Inherited Immunity

Inherited (inborn) immunity or susceptibility to disease can be confused with environmental factors. For example, comparisons are being made between the prevalence of tuberculosis in negroes compared to white Europeans and North Americans, suggesting a greater susceptibility in negroes. Tuberculosis, however, is known to be associated with poverty, malnutrition and overcrowding, so it may be these factors that contribute more and not an inherited predisposition to the disease. Evidence of inherited immunity has come from population studies and has suggested that susceptibility to poliomyelitis may be an inherited characteristic. Studies in twins have shown that for monozygotic twins (identical) if the first twin contracts tuberculosis then the second twin is more likely to also contract the disease when compared to second twins of dizygotic twins (non-identical). The frequency of infection of the second of dizygotic twins is similar to that for other brothers and sisters (siblings). In this type of immunity or susceptibility the genetic structure has a determining influence.

Acquired Immunity

In this type of immunity the body produces or receives antibodies against a specific micro-organism or its products. This may be obtained naturally or artificially.

Natural Immunity. This type of immunity may be obtained in two ways. Firstly there is the immunity which a newborn infant possesses. This is obtained from its mother during the course of development in the uterus as antibodies circulating in the mother's blood can cross the placenta to the developing foetus. The immunity which is transmitted to the foetus will reflect the exposure to disease naturally or the artificial acquisition of immunity by the mother. This naturally-acquired immunity of the infant is not, however, longlasting, generally disappearing by the age of six months, at which time the infant will depend on its own mechanism for producing antibodies. Maternal antibodies are also available to the infant in its early weeks of life through breast-feeding (Kilzinger 1979: 18). The mother's milk contains antibodies and in particular a specific antibody which helps protect the infant against bacterial invasion through its gastrointestinal wall. Thus, breast-feeding is not just simply a 'fad' which is promoted by paediatricians and obstetricians but has a vitally important role to play (Reeder, Mastroianni and Martin 1980: 476-7)

The second method of acquiring natural immunity is through direct contact with the disease. This type of acquired immunity may be associated with obvious clinical manifestations of the disease, but in some cases inapparent infection may occur which has the same effect, namely the production of antibodies but no obvious clinical signs. Natural immunity is important in the overall prevention of disease, as this increases the proportion of the population who are immune. Natural immunity may not be permanent and though mumps or chicken pox may confer life-long immunity, exposure to the common cold or influenza confers only limited immunity.

Artificial Immunity.   This process confers immunity by either provoking the production of antibodies (active immunity) or by the giving of antibodies (passive immunity). The process is termed immunisation and the choice of active or passive immunisation depends on the circumstances in which prevention is required.

Passive immunity is used when there is a need to protect individuals against the possibility of them contracting the disease during an outbreak and where the individual is known not to have previously been exposed to the disease and has no antibodies. In these circumstances immunity may be conferred by giving an injection of animal or human serum or human gammaglobulin, all of which are known to contain the requisite antibody, either obtained from direct infection or artificial inducement. The potent source of antibody is human gammaglobulin, which is the fraction of the sera containing antibodies. The use of human gammaglobulin has proved successful as a prophylactic measure during outbreaks of serum hepatitis, conferring immunity to those who have been exposed or need to be exposed because of their particular job, but who have not developed their own immunity. Passive immunity has the disadvantage of only conferring immunity for a short period of time but in addition the process may interfere with the individual's own defence mechanism, inhibiting antibody production.

Active immunity does not produce an immediate effect, taking at least three to four weeks to build up the levels of antibodies. The process of active immunity depends upon the challenge to the body's defence mechanism of live, killed or products from the specific micro-organism to stimulate the production of antibodies. This procedure comes under the generic title of immunisation.

Immunisation

Immunisation is a primary preventive measure, in that the process aims to protect an individual from developing clinical manifestations of disease when challenged by the micro-organism or its products; or to modify the actual disease process reducing its clinical effect. Not all artificially-induced immune response gives 100 per cent protection against a specific micro-organism. Measles may occur clinically in children who have received measles vaccine, though the clinical symptoms are much reduced. The cause of this modification in the immune response may be multifactorial. Certain preparations (vaccines) used to induce the artificial immune response require careful handling and may lose their potency if mishandled or stored improperly. In addition, however, the individual may have a deficient immune response mechanism and fail to produce antibodies, or the micro-organism's virulence may have altered and so the vaccine is no longer fully protective.

The immune response, as indicated previously, takes three to four weeks to reach a maximum effect following the introduction of the vaccine. This effect then may gradually wane so that repeated challenges may be required to produce high and persistent levels. These have the effect of not only increasing the amount of antibody produced but also the duration of its stay in circulation. These findings have led to schedules of immunisation against various infectious diseases being prepared for children. Table 9.2 outlines some of the schedules used in England and Wales for children.

Table 9.2: England and Wales: Summary of Immunisation Schedules for Children Aged 0-16 years

Age	Disease(s) against which immunisation is offered
3 months	Diphtheria, whooping cough, tetanus and polio (1st dose)
4-5 months	Diphtheria, whooping cough, tetanus and polio (2nd dose)
8-9 months	Diphtheria, whooping cough, tetanus and polio (3rd dose)
1-2 years	Measles
4-5 years	Diphtheria, tetanus and polio (pre-school booster)
11-13 years	Tuberculosis (BCG) after ascertaining state of immunity
12-13 years	Rubella (german measles) girls only
15-16 years	Tetanus and polio (booster before leaving school)

Source: Department of Health and Social Security *CMO(78)15*, HMSO, London.

Within the schedules there is provision for 'booster' immunisations. These boosters are included to ensure a high level of antibody against certain diseases, for example polio and tetanus. To ensure immunity to some diseases reimmunisation is suggested at periods as close as every three years; for people working in particular industries, for example agriculture, booster injections against tetanus are proposed every five years.

The type of vaccine used in inducing immunity varies according to the disease. Three main types of vaccine are commonly used: vaccines containing live micro-organisms; vaccines containing killed micro-organisms; and vaccines containing the products of micro-organisms (toxins).

Vaccines Containing Live Micro-organisms.   In the preparation of these vaccines, the micro-organisms (bacteria or virus) used are either of low virulence or they have been attenuated, that is their harmful effect has been reduced but they will still provoke an antibody response in an individual. Live bacteria are used in the preparation of the vaccine used for producing immunity to tuberculosis, but the organism itself is derived from a bovine tubercle bacillus, of low virulence in man but producing an antibody response to the human tubercle bacillus. In the vaccine used against polio, live viruses of the three antigenic types of polio virus are used. The viruses have been attenuated and the mutant viruses have lost their power to produce paralysis but retain their power to grow in the human intestine and provide the necessary antigenic stimulus to give an antibody response. Other examples of live attenuated vaccines containing viruses include measles and rubella (german measles).

Vaccines Containing Killed or Inactivated Micro-organisms.   In the preparation of these vaccines heat or phenol is used to kill the micro-organism, which still retains its power to provide an antibody response. Killed bacteria are used in the preparation of the vaccine T.A.B. which produces antibodies against typhoid, paratyphoid A and paratyphoid B. Inactivated viruses are used in the preparation of vaccines against influenza and rabies.

Vaccines Containing Products of Micro-organisms.   The development of these vaccines, producing antitoxic immunity, became essential because in some diseases it is not the organism which is the main factor in producing the clinical manifestations of the disease, but their products — toxins. To counter the clinical effect of the toxins, vaccines have been produced using the toxin but modifying it by combining it with formalin to give a product termed a toxoid.

This modified preparation will induce the body's defence mechanism to produce antitoxins which will counter the effect of the toxin produced by the micro-organism, should it invade the individual. The two major diseases where prevention has been of value using toxoid preparations to produce antitoxic immunity are diphtheria and tetanus.

The development of immunisation procedures has enabled a number of infectious diseases to be controlled and hence offer to a population the possibility of primary prevention of the diseases and their eventual eradication, such as occurred with smallpox. The next disease which the World Health Organisation has indicated is of major importance is poliomyelitis and now a worldwide campaign is being followed to eradicate this particular disease. Eradication, however, depends on high levels of immunity in the population, conversely epidemics indicate high susceptibility and low immunity. The level of immunity in a population for any particular disease depends on the proportion of that population who have acquired immunity. Artificially-acquired immunity has, as shown, limitations in terms of the length of time the immunity remains. Passive immunity acquired through the injection of antibodies also has a limited lifespan of weeks or months. Artificially-induced active immunity takes time to build up and may require repeated challenges to produce high levels of circulatory antibodies which will remain viable. Table 9.3 outlines the different vaccine preparations. Thus, there are technical problems in the maintenance of adequately high levels and achievement of primary prevention may involve a number of factors, for example education, engineering and legislation.

Table 9.3: Examples of Different Types of Vaccine Preparations against Diseases

Live	
Bacterial	Tuberculosis
Viral	Measles, polio, rubella
Killed or inactivated	
Bacterial	Typhoid fever
Viral	Influenza, rabies
Rickettsial	Typhus fever
Products (Toxins)	Diphtheria, tetanus
Used to induce ACTIVE immunity	
Immunoglobulins	
Normal	Hepatitis B, measles
Specific	Rabies, tetanus, smallpox
Anti-D (Rho)	Prevents rhesus negative mothers forming antibodies against rhesus positive foetus
Used to give PASSIVE immunity	

Non-infectious Disease Prevention

So far in this chapter we have dealt specifically with infectious diseases but acute non-infectious diseases also are as important in the preventive policies of any government. Because of the vast range of non-infectious diseases within the community there needs to be a constant review of what is actually happening to the pattern of disease, and this has been discussed in Chapter 2. For example, evidence has shown that the mortality from cancer of the lung in women is still continuing to rise, whilst that in men has begun to fall. Cardiovascular disease, and in particular coronary heart disease, is known to be a major cause of morbidity and mortality in England and Wales, and the association between cigarette smoking and coronary heart disease is now well-established. For other diseases, for example the cancers, attention is now being focused on occupational groups who may be at risk and mention has already been made of the relationship between asbestos workers and the development of cancer of the lung in later life.

The epidemiological investigation of the trends in disease pattern has suggested that for some diseases the apparent increase may be due to improved diagnosis, but in other cases it may be an actual increase in the amount of the disease occurring. Other diseases have however shown a decline. For example in England and Wales acute appendicitis has declined both in mortality and incidence over the past 40 years, as reported by Donnan and Lambert (1976: 26-8).

The understanding, therefore, of the epidemiology of non-infectious diseases is becoming an increasingly important aspect of our knowledge in terms of trying to assess the possible preventive measures that may be undertaken. Alteration in disease pattern, as suggested by Barker (1982: 18-20) is that non-infectious diseases themselves do not occur at an unchanging rate from year to year but there are upsurges, declines and fluctuations. Thus the pattern of disease changes all the time and for the most part the changes cannot always be predicted. Barker quotes that the number of suicides by poisoning with domestic coal gas increased sharply in England and Wales in 1958, but subsequently there has been a decline, as indicated in Chapter 7 (p. 82), due to change in the type of gas entering the home. Similarly we know that there are changes in the pattern of accident attendances at accident departments during a particular year. Thus, the prevention of non-infectious diseases is not as simple as that of infectious diseases, though this should not deter the epidemiologist from looking at the distribution and determinants of their cause.

Factors Involved in Primary Prevention

In discussing primary prevention and the factors involved, the three that are outlined – education, legislation and engineering – are as applicable to infectious as non-infectious disease. The principle behind all three is to try and prevent disease from occurring within a community and an outline is given of the role and function of each.

Education. To maintain the momentum within a population towards primary prevention education is an essential feature. Schools and colleges are involved in this educative process through a wide variety of subjects in their curriculum. This may include such aspects as simple hygiene, use of immunisation to prevent disease, factors about health and its maintenance, and the production of ill-health through self-inflicted disease arising from smoking and alcohol. These activities are often brought together under the generic title of health education and are primary preventive methods in relation to disease control. This principle of health education can be extended to the place of work and as the Department of Health and Social Security (1976) indicated, prevention and health are everybody's business. This implies, therefore, that people should be aware of the problems and educate themselves to the dangers surrounding them.

Engineering. This is an important factor in primary prevention of disease that includes not only engineering methods to reduce hazards in industry but also laboratory engineering to investigate new vaccines. One might also include within this engineering in terms of epidemiological investigations, that is to determine the distribution and determinants of disease in man. These may very well involve using laboratory techniques. Examples of primary preventive measures in industrial engineering have been those to remove hazardous products and to create a safe environment, for example air filters and dust extraction units. But engineering relies, as does education, on an understanding of the causal factor or factors before the engineering can become a major influence and a primary preventive measure.

Legislation. Legislation has been used successfully in primary prevention, particularly in the industrial field through the Health and Safety at Work (etc) Act 1974. Much of the legislation is now aimed at preventing disease and, in particular, accidents. Legislation has, however, been used in this country in respect of infectious disease control, enabling quarantine regulations to be enforced. Smallpox vaccination was a legal requirement in England and Wales, and in respect of tuberculosis control powers still exist to enforce removal of patients to hospital for care. Compulsory immunisation against infectious disease is, however, no longer practised in England and Wales and education is preferred, but legislation does, however, exist in other countries, for example the United States, and parents there have to show certificates of immunisation of their children before they can start school.

Prevention of disease, therefore, is a complex process and, perhaps unfortunately, curative treatment has become synonymous with prevention of disease. In this chapter prevention has been described at two levels, of which curative medicine is the second level, perhaps suggesting a failure. That modern medicine and nursing can eradicate and prevent pathological consequences of disease is not questioned, but the fact remains that to practise these skills the patient has to have the disease. Prevention of disease is concerned with the ultimate eradication of disease from a population and this means preventing the disease from occurring in the individuals who make up that population. To identify the cause of the disease, as well as the distribution, so that primary prevention may become possible, even if this may take a long time as it did for smallpox, must, therefore, still be the epidemiologist's primary concern.

10 PLANNING FOR HEALTH CARE FOR A COMMUNITY

In this chapter the idea of planning health services will be considered and discussed with particular relevance to the role of epidemiology (Knox 1979). Epidemiology established itself mainly in infectious disease and has subsequently tackled problems of chronic disease and disability which are now the outstanding health problems throughout most of the Western world. In recent years epidemiology has moved into the field of health care planning. Planning has been defined as 'the selection of the best available alternatives to achieve specific goals', or 'the exercise of intelligence to deal with facts and situations as they are and finally to solve problems'. Planning, and planners, have come in for some hard knocks in recent years, but few would seriously advocate that organised attempts to improve health services should now be abandoned; what is now required is more discussion on how best to plan. Perhaps the achievements of planning have not been sufficiently recognised by society in general and by health professionals in particular. Without planning nearby hospitals would all want to have their own cardiac and neurosurgical units, with the spending of more money and with probably less satisfactory treatment for the patients involved. This indeed does happen in some parts of the world and it is partly because, in Britain, we have got used to some planning that we are perhaps not sufficiently aware of what can happen without it. The accusation that the National Health Service is expensive is certainly not supported by international comparisons. There are problems in comparing expenditures between countries, but the use of the percentage of the gross national product (GNP) spent on health services is generally a valid comparison. The UK still devotes a smaller proportion of its gross national product to health compared with many other countries. In 1975 most Western countries spent between 6.9 per cent (Switzerland) and 9.4 per cent (West Germany) of their GNP on health whereas Britain spent only 5.2 per cent. It is still spending below 6 per cent of its GNP on health services, yet no one is prevented from using the service by lack of means. However, as discussed in Chapter 7, Section 2, not all who would benefit from treatment are able to receive it and others may have to wait for considerable periods.

The Role of Epidemiology

It is important to distinguish clearly between planning for health and planning medical care services. Epidemiology has an important role in health planning. It also has a more specific role in the planning of medical care services. The distinction between these two aspects of planning is important as health problems can be tackled either through attempting to organise better services for their treatment or by attempting prevention. Prevention often involves other aspects of social policy, many of which are not usually considered as policies for health. Also public health measures, as for example the provision of clean water and sanitation, as well as public education and legislation, on such things as accidents, nutrition and clear air, are important in prevention. Prevention of disease may also be enhanced by taxation policies. The evaluation of the effectiveness of taxation on such things as cigarettes and alcohol and the effectiveness of health education campaigns requires the use of epidemiology, because such studies must be conducted in defined populations or in samples of such populations. There is no doubt that much of our present standards of health, and increasing expectation of life, are associated with the prevention of diseases, both by public health measures, legislation and education as well as the increasing standards of living that have occurred through most of the last two centuries.

In considering the role of epidemiology in health, let us consider the example of cigarette smoking. As a habit it is almost confined to the last hundred years, but is one that has done enormous damage to the health of the population during this time, causing much illness and mortality. About a fifth of all deaths in England and Wales are now thought to be directly attributable to cigarette smoking. Epidemiologists have surveyed both the smoking habit in different population groups and the resulting diseases which this causes. Twenty years ago there was little social class difference in the prevalence of cigarette smokers in the population. However, since the first reports of the dangers of cigarette smoking, the decline in the population of smokers has been very much greater in social classes I (professional) and II (intermediate) than in the other social classes. This emerging difference in the proportion of cigarette smokers between social classes presumably has been a result of health education of some sort. As well as a change in numbers there has also been a change in the type of cigarette smoked. Since the late 1950s, there has been a marked increase in the proportion of filter-tipped cigarettes and a corresponding decline in the proportion of plain cigarettes smoked. It is, however, difficult to know how people get their information on such topics and why some act on it while others do not. This is a complex field and while it is obvious that more health education is needed, the type of education required is less obvious and money spent on health education should be accompanied by money to allow evaluation of the effect of the health education. However, health education is probably not the only factor at work in reducing cigarette consumption. There have been a number of restrictions on advertising and in some countries there is now a total ban in operation on cigarette advertising. A number of studies in the United Kingdom have shown that the consumption of cigarettes is related to their price. When the price goes up (and this is largely owing to increases in taxation) the consumption falls, although this effect may sometimes be only temporary. While most Chancellors of the Exchequer probably regard taxation of tobacco as largely a means of increasing revenue, it does have a very important part to play in promoting the health of the population. Indeed this role has now been recognised and used, as there is a new differential taxation such that those cigarettes with lower tar yields are now cheaper than cigarettes with higher yields. This differential tax, as well as the health education, may be the reason why many more people are changing over to lower tar cigarettes. There is little information yet on how much safer such cigarettes are but such evidence is beginning to emerge and it is reasonable to expect that they are less dangerous than those with high tar yields. Further, individuals smoking low tar cigarettes may find it easier to stop and therefore may be more susceptible to health education in the future.

Epidemiology and Health Care Planning

Recently epidemiologists have become increasingly involved in the use of epidemiology in the planning of medical care services. One of the reasons for this is probably the rapid increase in the use of data handling methods, including computers, which provide information which the epidemiologist and planners can use. Another factor that has led to the use of epidemiologists in planning services has been the increasing technical complexity and cost of medicine and the increasing realisation that resources are in fact always limited when compared with the ideal. This has led to the demand for the rational use of our existing resources in the way that would give the greatest benefit. When it is realised and accepted that it is no longer possible to provide everything, it becomes desirable to use services as efficiently as possible.

For epidemiologists to become involved in health care planning, they must have a general idea of how planning is done. A model of the planning cycle is shown in Figure 10.1. Planning consists of a series of steps which are followed in a more or less systematic way. It is perhaps logical to begin this cycle with the identification of the problems and then the formulation of objectives. It is then usual to consider a number of possible alternative policies by which these objectives might be achieved. Unless it is deliberately decided to investigate several alternatives for research purposes, it is usual to select just one of these policies and to create from it the operational plan. This plan is then discussed and implemented and, following its implementation, there should be an evaluation of the extent to which the operational plan has in fact met the stated objectives. From this evaluation there comes the identification of new problems, the character of which will of course depend upon the success or otherwise of the initial plan.

Figure 10.1: The Planning Cycle

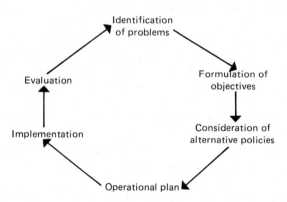

Undoubtedly at first sight many workers in the health field would regard the figure of the planning cycle (Figure 10.1) as being a very academic approach to what they would regard as a very practical problem. They may, for instance, query whether it is necessary to go into details with such things as the formulation of objectives. However, most people would now agree that it is necessary to do some form of evaluation of all aspects of health service (see Chapter 11). It is in practice not possible to evaluate anything unless one has clearly stated objectives. Evaluation, in fact, is the process of relating the outcome of the service to the stated objectives. If there are no objectives one cannot measure whether they have been achieved! It is, therefore, best to regard both planning and evaluation as part of a continuous interactive process and hence a circle, as shown in the figure. This monitoring must usually be continuous, or at least attempted from time to time, as circumstances may well change and the original validations, or even the original objectives, may no longer be appropriate. If one accepts this cycle of evaluation and planning, it follows that the epidemiologist must be involved at all stages of the planning process. It is only then that they will be able to increase their usefulness, which is basically their particular contribution to the evaluation of the service. In practice, it is extremely difficult, and often impossible, to try and evaluate a service without some input into the planning of that service. Evaluation then can rarely be done in isolation. Just as the epidemiologist must be involved in planning, so too must the planners and other groups of health professionals understand the role of the epidemiologist and what he is doing.

Gathering and Utilising Necessary Information

One of the epidemiologist's contributions to the planning cycle will be the identification of sources of information which can be used to identify problems and to formulate objectives. Within the health service there are a number of routine sources of information which can be used for these purposes. This information concerns such activities as number of hospital discharges and information on manpower, and is then often combined with information from other sources, particularly demographic information about the health district or region. Much of this information comes from the national census. There is information available which shows, by age and sex, the number of people living in different parts of the country. As we have already described, the prevalence of many diseases is closely related to age. As a whole the age structure of the population in the country is changing, and is doing so even more rapidly in some smaller areas. There is also movement of the population from one area to another so that some areas have an increased total population whereas others have a decline in total numbers. Changes are particularly important when we consider the proportion of the elderly in the population. The number of people over 65 years of age in England and Wales increased from 1.7 million in 1901 to about 8 million in 1981. Again, considering those over the age of 65 years, the proportion in the population has increased by over a fifth in the last 15 years. Current projections suggest that the corresponding growth in the next 15 years will be considerably less but that, amongst the elderly, the proportion of those who are aged 75 or over will continue to increase. As prevalence of a number of diseases increases markedly with increasing age, the age structure of the population is a very important factor in the demand for health services. For example, the proportion of individuals aged 85 years and over in a geriatric bed is 10-15 times the proportion of individuals aged 65-74. Even when one looks at acute medical and acute surgical beds, the bed occupation rates per thousand of the elderly, are very much more in those aged 85 and over than they are in those aged 65-74 years.

From the above considerations it is possible to plan the Health Service for changes in the age structure in the population, using population projections which are available for various areas for a number of years into the future. While many population projections which involve the birth rate have been inaccurate in the past, projections concerning the elderly, because there has been little change in mortality rates in this age group, have been relatively accurate. It should, therefore, be possible to try and plan health services so as to cope with the differing demands placed upon the health services by population changes.

Whenever possible such plans should be as specific as the information allows. For instance, in considering orthopaedic services, the rates for fracture of the hip are known in different age groups. This is a condition which has a particularly marked increase with age and population projections can be used to calculate the number of fractures which health services will be likely to deal with in future years. One necessarily makes the assumption here that the age-specifc rates for fractures of the hip will not change much over time. Such assumptions are not always justified, but are perhaps less likely to show important changes than are the techniques used for dealing with the condition. In considering a fractured hip, it would be necessary to plan not only the number of operating theatres and operating staff that would be required, but also to make assumptions about the length of stay in hospital in each case and any future changes that may occur in the average length of stay. In the past, for a wide variety of conditions, the average stay in hospital has been decreasing and this in itself, if the trend continues, will have an effect on the number of beds required. Such calculations frequently show the need for increasing resources to run the Health Service to make available similar provisions of care over a period of time to the whole population. This is due to the fact that over recent years the increasing proportion of the elderly, and especially of the

85+ age group, has led to a greater demand and need for health services. In making these predictions about future trends, calculations should be made using local information, because many of the trends discussed above are overall national trends. It is important to remember that there are very considerable variations in different parts of the country.

The example considered here has been the use of population projections for the elderly. Information at the other end of the age spectrum can be used for planning obstetric services and for infant and child health care. However, as already mentioned, our predictions for changes in birth rate are very much less accurate than are the predictions for the proportion of the elderly in the population. This makes the planning of the required number of obstetric beds a much more difficult problem. In addition, there are considerable variations in the length of hospital stay after delivery and the proportion of all babies that are born in hospital (which will depend partly on the proportion of babies that are born to mothers of various parities) may also vary considerably. When it comes to school health services there are much more accurate population predictions for five years before the time.

Implementing Change

In planning health services it is often necessary to make a critical study of the beneficial effects and the efficiency with which the present services are being run. This research is necessary but is often seen as threatening by others involved in the Health Service. It may be seen, quite correctly, as an attempt at organisational change and this often arouses suspicion that some of those employed in the Health Service may be directly or indirectly affected one way or another. There may be reduced responsibility, more work, or less work, because of the changes suggested. However, the objective of this planning is to make a more effective and efficient Health Service, to improve the health of the population as a whole and, in particular, to make a better outcome in the case of those having specific treatments. This necessitates that those evaluating the service, and hence those often seen to be criticising it, are accepted and trusted by those involved in patient-care and also those involved in the administration of the service. An understanding of epidemiology by all health care professionals and Health Service administrators is one way to try and reduce such frictions between interested groups, to the benefit of the health of the population in the future. This is required for the new multidisciplinary approach to health care planning.

11 EVALUATION

What is Evaluation?

Evaluation is the process which attempts to measure whether the stated objectives of a defined programme of activity are being achieved. In this chapter evaluation will be discussed with specific reference to health care in its broadest context (service and/or treatment). The argument could be put forward that if those people involved in the provision of health care have been properly trained and have accredited qualifications, then the services provided should be satisfactory and meeting their objectives and evaluation is unnecessary. This argument makes certain assumptions, for example: that there is a clear agreed objective for the service and that people are aware of it; that the most efficient method(s) are being used to provide the service; and that people who require the service are obtaining it.

Evaluation as a process therefore attempts to measure how far the service (or treatment) is meeting the stated objectives, but also may reveal alternative methods of providing the service. It thus forms an integral part of the 'planning process' which is described in Chapter 10. Just as planning of services requires the planner(s) to state the objectives for that service, so the person evaluating those services must state the specific areas (objectives) which will be covered during the evaluation process.

The objectives set by the evaluator are generally considered at two levels: global – the overall assessment of a service; and specific – a particular part of the service.

Global Evaluation. In this process of evaluation the investigator attempts to measure whether the objectives set for the health services in relation to a defined population, for example a District Health Authority, are being or have been achieved. The evaluator would require a definition of the District Health Authority's objectives in respect of the services it is providing. The evaluator would then have to decide how refined the evaluation process was to be.

Obviously the evaluation of an Authority's entire services would be a major undertaking and would require considerable resources. Such a study would require complex data collection systems, computer facilities for analysis of the data, and skilled personnel to carry out the review. This example is perhaps extreme, but even the assessment of just one service, for example the Authority's 'Obstetric Services' would be within the category of a global evaluation. Such an evaluation would have to look not only at how the service was being provided physically, but outcome, in terms of such measures as perinatal mortality (stillbirths and deaths within the first seven days of life, expressed as a proportion of total births) and abnormal deliveries and compare these, where possible, against local or nationally accepted standards or norms. Thus a simple analysis of the component parts of an obstetric service indicates how complex an evaluation process would be on a global basis. Even with local or nationally agreed standards set as objectives these might only be for certain aspects of the service. The remainder would have to be evaluated against, perhaps, non-numeric objectives, making the process more complex. Where there are accepted standards then a more restricted (specific) evaluation may be possible.

Specific Evaluation.   This type of evaluation is used when only a part of the service is being studied, and particularly where there are accepted standards of performance which act as the objective(s) to be achieved. Using perinatal mortality as an example, the objective set for part of the obstetric service is to achieve a perinatal mortality rate equal to or better than the national rate. This rate is measurable and can therefore be used to evaluate how far that particular objective of the service has been achieved, or if it differs what were the possible causes.

In this more limited approach, the process of evaluation becomes easier and where possible should be an integral part of the service when it is established. In some circumstances this ideal is not possible, the service having been in operation for some time. In these instances the evaluator may have to collect data (information) retrospectively or prospectively as part of an ongoing study. In both cases the data collection must be as accurate and representative of what is occurring throughout the service being evaluated.

In a study of accident and emergency services, and an evaluation of the provision of facilities for children attending accident and emergency units, the evaluator may need to collect data for a whole year. Evidence has shown that there are variations in the number of attendances of children aged 0-15 years, with peaks in the months of July and August, related to school holidays. Home accidents have been shown to be associated with these peaks of hospital attendance (Department of Trade 1981: 30).

As mentioned previously the ideal planning of a service would incorporate a built-in evaluation mechanism. An example where such a mechanism was applied can be found in the introduction of five-day care units. In such units patients are admitted between Monday and Friday and in practice the ward closes on Friday afternoon. All patients must therefore be discharged *home* by that time. If a patient is too ill then that patient would have to be transferred to another ward. This transfer represents in effect a 'failed case', that is, one of the objectives of the system, discharging all patients home, has not been achieved.

Five-day care units have been in operation in a number of centres and have been described by Longston and Young (1973: 528-31) and Burgess, Chant and Beschi (1978: 427-8). Burgess *et al* (1978) described the policies for the unit, which in effect are objectives. Thus the evaluator could use the policies as the criteria against which to evaluate the overall achievements of the unit or part of it. The process of evaluation involves the use of different methods, some scientifically-based (data collection and measurement) some less scientifically-based (opinion), this latter group being generally less acceptable.

Limits to Evaluation. While this chapter sets out to show the need for and method of evaluation, the present limits to evaluation must be appreciated. While health services always *should* have objectives, it is not always possible to measure whether these are being achieved. There is an obvious tendency to measure things that are easy to measure but we must not ignore things that are important but difficult, perhaps at present impossible to measure. But health professionals should always be seeking ways to evaluate treatments and services. As Chapter 7, Section 2 showed, patients with kidney disease are now dying because treatment facilities are not available. Health professionals and management have a duty to assess all their activities in order to provide the best overall service that the available resources will allow.

Methods of Evaluation

Any method used in the process of evaluation must be accurate, valid and repeatable. The evaluator would, where possible, prefer to be able to use at all times scientific measurements which have been well tried and generally accepted. This may not always be possible and less reliable methods may have, because of expediency, to be accepted. Three basic methods of evaluation can be identified: opinion – subjective and based on personal assessment; descriptive — uses scientific measurement; experimental — establishes scientific tests and analyses data from these.

Opinion

Opinion is a subjective method of evaluation and may be misleading, particularly where the evaluator is familiar with the service. In these circumstances the evaluator makes a subjective assessment, perhaps using some scale such as poor, good or excellent. Such an evaluation can be biased either by lack of knowledge and understanding, or by expert knowledge of the situation. Similarly, if the evaluator asks for opinions, unless there is some structured format the value of the findings may be of little benefit. Opinion does not involve direct measurement such as blood pressure, birth rate, but there are methods of utilising opinion in a structured way through the use of questionnaires, and these methods are described in the book by Moser and Kalton (1972). Two types of opinion are quoted by evaluators, expert and non-expert.

Expert Opinion.   Where the evaluator is unable to carry out scientific assessment of the service, expert opinion may be sought to try and reach some conclusion. As suggested in the previous paragraph this may lead to bias in the views expressed, either intentionally or more probably unintentionally, because only certain aspects of the service may be highlighted, namely the most favourable. Personal opinion, even expert opinion, is likely to be biased by particular cases or events, which may be unrepresentative, but because of personal involvement with a patient are likely to unduly colour the individual's opinion. The patient who develops a rare complication with a drug, or a child brain-damaged from a vaccine, may discourage the caring professional from recommending such drugs or vaccines in the future. While such tragic events should not be ignored, in any evaluation, they should be placed in a wider statistical perspective of risk. This means that most individual health professionals do not see enough cases to assess the risks of rare events and information from any individuals must be pooled together to obtain meaningful results. In the case of vaccine damage of children, it makes little sense for some professionals to stop using the vaccine if they have experience of brain-damage while others continue to use it, saying in their experience it is completely safe. What is needed is a sound assessment of risks and benefits which is not possible within the experience of the professional.

An example of a possibly biased evaluation of a maternity service could arise from seeking the opinion of the local midwives providing a service to a general practitioner obstetric unit based in a community hospital servicing a small town. The opinions given may suggest a service which is less stressful to the patient than the consultant unit, the mother is cared for by the practitioner who has carried out her ante-natal care and relatives can visit easily. The impression given is of a high quality service with a firm conviction, based on long experience, that there is a very low perinatal mortality rate. However, what may be overlooked is the proportion of women who, in the course of labour, develop complications and have to be transferred to the consultant unit at a District General Hospital, a proportion which may exceed 20 per cent of all booked cases. Omission of this data would give a misleading impression, so that even expert opinion may be unintentionally biased if there are no measureable objectives or standards.

Non-expert Opinion. The most obvious example of non-expert opinion is *public opinion* and this is often used by newspapers to assess how the public may vote at an election or react to proposed changes in legislation. Public opinion about matters of health and safety have been studied and indicate the lack of knowledge which the public have about a health matter and yet express firm opinions. In a study by the Wessex Positive Health Team (1980) into the possibility of promoting seat belt wearing by car occupants, members of the public were asked to state why they did not wear a seat belt. Whilst about 50 per cent could be grouped within the headings: forgetful, not developed the habit, 9 per cent said that seat belts would trap them in the car in the event of a crash and 8 per cent said that it was the fear of being burnt to death, implying the seat belt would prevent them getting out of the car.

Studies had, prior to 1980, been carried out by the Transport and Road Research Laboratory into the protection that seat belts afforded and Hobbs (1981) published information about the benefits that the earlier research had shown. Whilst they did not prevent all injury, they considerably reduced the effect, and the distortion of the car's body was the cause of people being trapped, not the seat belts. With regard to the risk of fire, Hobbs (1978: 13-14) indicated that the risk of being trapped inside a vehicle where fire or submersion in water occurs, is very small, estimated at 1 in 1000. Lack of knowledge of the facts can bias public opinion and hence their attitude towards a service or preventive measure.

For some evaluation it is necessary to use patients' opinion, and this can be achieved by the use of questionnaires, properly designed and tested. Minear and Lucente (1979: 1061-5) carried out a study using questionnaires to evaluate the service they were providing for patients who had undergone laryngectomy for cancer of the larynx. From their study they were able to obtain information indicating areas where objectives were not achieved and assumptions about the value of certain procedures were shown to be incorrect. A study by Shim and Williams (1980: 11-13) evaluated patients' assessment of their disability from asthma attacks compared to physicians'. This study collected not only patient opinion but also used clinical measurement, and showed that patients were superior in their assessment of disability compared to the physician. Thus, evaluation using opinion in a structured way can be of benefit, but unstructured opinions without knowledge can be misleading.

Descriptive Methods

In this type of study of evaluation indices of measurement form an integral part of the study process. This allows data (information) to be collected in a numerical format capable of detailed analysis. As the title suggests descriptive methods describe and measure what has occurred over time and assess whether the achievements of the service or treatment meet the objectives. Two types of studies are commonly used, before and after studies, and longitudinal studies.

Before and After Studies.   As the name implies these types of studies involve the measurement of a service over one period of time and then for a further period after some change has occurred, that is, a new objective has been proposed. This implies, however, that the experiment, that is, the change, could have been uncontrolled, but in most studies this is not the case and the change is deliberate.

An example of this type of study occurred when local authorities changed from the policy of full physical medical examinations to one of a medical questionnaire and selected medical examinations for employees entering their service. The objective of the change was to reduce the amount of time spent by doctors examining large numbers of 'fit people' (healthy) through the use of a medical questionnaire which each new employee had to complete. The doctor examined the replies contained in the questionnaires and if there was no evidence of previous illness necessitating further investigation, then that potential employee could be declared fit for employment. Where there was doubt then the doctor could ask for further details and see the person concerned.

Evaluation of this change would require a measurement of the proportion of people found unfit by the two systems and whether there had been any increase after the change in the sickness absence rates, or in the number of people who had to be discharged from employment because of ill-health, which should have been found at their first application for a post through the use of the medical questionnaire.

Longitudinal Studies. These types of studies are used particularly in evaluating a new form of treatment, though are applicable to health services. The evaluation requires some comparable treatment information to be available so that the new treatment can be assessed against other existing treatments. Such studies have been carried out in examining different types of treatment for cancers for example breast cancer. The results of the study may be expressed as the survival time, for example five year survival.

Other studies may evaluate alternative strategies for care, for particular conditions. In a study by Morris, Ward and Handyside (1968: 681-5) they compared the outcome of patients who had had the operative procedure inguinal herniorrhaphy. Some patients were discharged home the same day whilst others remained in hospital for 10 days. The study compared the outcomes of the two groups of patients over time within given criteria (objectives). No difference was found and the conclusions could be drawn that day surgical care for the repair of inguinal hernia was comparable in its outcome to that of the traditional ten-day hospital care.

In these types of studies the evaluator has a number of measurements that he can use to allow him to compare different treatments or changes in health service pattern. Such measures may include case fatality rates; readmission rates; standardised mortality ratios; and survival rates. In some of these studies the division between a descriptive method and an experimental method became blurred.

Experimental Methods

This group of studies used in the evaluation of services or treatments, as in descriptive studies, makes use of data and sets out to collect data to help in the evaluation process. There are a number of different types of experimental methods which may be used in evaluation and four are outlined.

Natural Experiments. In this situation the evaluator takes no participative action but observes and records data about changes and what effect these have had. An example of a natural experiment where evaluation of the benefits of change were measured was that concerning the relationship between hard and soft water supplies and mortality from ischaemic heart disease. Observations suggested that there might be an association between the mortality rate from ischaemic heart disease and hard water, there being an apparently lower mortality in populations having hard water compared to populations living in soft water areas. Obviously this difference could have been due to other factors, but by chance some previously soft water areas had had their water supplies hardened before this apparent association was reported. By examining the mortality rate in the areas of previously soft water which had been hardened (before and after study) the evidence suggested a decrease in the mortality in these areas from ischaemic heart disease. There are obviously a number of other aspects which need consideration and these are discussed more fully in the paper relating to this subject by Gardner (1973: 421-40).

Other studies of a similar nature have involved the use of fluoride in water supplies and its effect on the prevalence of dental caries. Fluoride is known to have a protective effect and evidence has shown that where fluoride occurs naturally in high levels the prevalence of dental caries in children is lower compared to areas where there is a low level of fluoride. A similar finding has been found where fluoride has been deliberately introduced (not a natural experiment) and its evaluation has been reported by Rock, Gordon and Bradnock (1981: 61-6). Rock *et al.* were able to show that where fluoride had been introduced artificially into the water supplies which had previously had low levels, the prevalence of dental caries had reduced.

Randomised Trials.   This type of experimental method is used principally in the evaluation of clinical practice to compare two different forms of therapy or assess the effect of a new drug, using another drug as a control. This allows measurements to be taken and the data collected to be analysed and an objective evaluation to be carried out by com- parison. The use of randomised trials is complex, as outlined in Chapter 4, and depends upon the random allocation of patients to the different treatments being evaluated and, in the case of drugs, very specific con- trols to ensure that neither the patient nor the doctor knows which drug has been administered.

An example of a comparison between two treatments and the evalua- tion in terms of cost to the Health Service, was that carried out by Chant, Jones and Weddell (1972: 1188-91) relating to varicose veins. Patients were allocated either to surgical or injection (sclerosing) treat- ments randomly. The objectives of the evaluation related not only to cost of the service but patient satisfaction.

Randomised trials, however, have limitations, namely the results can only be related to the parameters within which the trial was carried out. For example, the route of administration of the drug (oral or injection), the dose and frequency of administration. In addition the measurements of the effects produced must be precisely recorded, whether this is by physical measurement or a structured questionnaire.

Non-randomised Trials. In this method of evaluation people with similar conditions are allocated (chosen) for one of two types of treatment. This may immediately introduce bias either on the part of the person allocating the patients or because the patients themselves know what treatment they are having compared to others, which may lead to dissatisfaction totally unrelated to the effect of the treatment. Where possible this type of trial should be avoided.

Operational Research. This is a specialised form of research requiring an understanding of mathematics, statistics and computing. Basically it is a technique whereby using mathematical data and changing parts of the data, the evaluator can examine what happens to the whole of the data. If this data is made to represent a certain form of treatment then obviously substituting change in treatment, predictions can be made as to whether this will be beneficial or not.

Operational research techniques have been used to examine health services and specific forms of treatment. West, Crosby and Jones (1974: 149-55) used this technique to evaluate the outcome of the treatment of patients with acute renal failure by dialysis or dialysis and transplantation.

Other Aspects of Evaluation

The various methods of evaluation described attempt to provide a framework within which the evaluator can work and base his findings where possible and preferably on scientifically collected data. When considering the results the evaluator will need to also consider these in relation to three criteria — efficacy, effectiveness and efficiency. These three terms are used quite precisely in epidemiological evaluation and are of importance in the overall evaluation.

Efficacy. This is interpreted as a measure of the extent to which a service or treatment alters the natural course (history) of a disease or the health of the population. That is, whether the service or treatment is actually beneficial or harmful. Thus, in the evaluation of a new vaccine for protection of a population against polio, the evaluator must be sure not only that the vaccine does what the manufacturers claim but it also is safe (i.e. does not produce cases of polio).

Effectiveness.   This is interpreted as measure of whether the service actually reaches or is available to those who need it. The effectiveness of the screening programme for cervical cancer in women has been mentioned in Chapter 8 and may be used as an example of a service which is not as effective as would be desirable following evaluation — the service does not reach large numbers of the 'at risk' population.

Efficiency.   This is interpreted as a measure of whether the service or treatment is being provided in the most inexpensive way possible. In looking at this criterion the cost must include not only the revenue costs (expenditure on manpower, drugs, lighting, heating) but also the capital costs, that is paying for the bricks and mortar.

Effectiveness and efficiency are closely linked. If the cost of the service rises then that service may have to be limited, reducing its effectiveness, but in doing so the benefit of that service may also be reduced within the population. Thus cost and benefit are linked and become another aspect of evaluation.

Cost and Benefit

The interrelationship between cost and benefit can be examined under the two headings: cost effectiveness and cost benefit.

Cost Effectiveness.   This method examines, as already outlined, the cost of undertaking a service or treatment in relation to the population who need it. Thus, cost effectiveness will examine the financial aspects of the service, that is expenditure. This expenditure will consist of both revenue and capital cost. For example, the cost effectiveness of a service would include the cost of labour, dressings, lighting and heating as well as any building or equipment. Obviously the evaluator would need to examine whether the service was being provided in the cheapest way possible and reaching the maximum number of people or whether there was possibly some other way.

Cost Benefit.   This method examines not only the cost in terms of service provision, but also whether those people receiving the treatment actually benefit from it, and considers the efficacy as well as the efficiency. It is because efficacy is often difficult to measure that cost benefit studies are more difficult than cost effectiveness studies.

The dividing line between evaluation and planning is blurred. Planning is concerned with setting objectives but must know within that process whether these objectives are met. This requires evaluation and within the framework of this process the evaluator may suggest alternatives — new plans which will have objectives. Evaluation brings to the Health Service an approach, scientifically based, to measure whether objectives are being met.

Without evaluation we have no way of knowing whether the health care services are achieving their objectives. Without objectives for the services then evaluation cannot be carried out. Without objective evaluation traditional patterns of care may remain often outmoded and without any scientific basis for their practice. This is not to say those new concepts necessarily prove to be more beneficial. A study and analysis of five-day care wards in England and Wales by Davies, Cliff and Waters (1981: 2118-19) indicated that some of these units were far from being used either efficiently or to their greatest potential. Evaluation is an integral part of planning services or treatment and should be built into the provision of any new service to ensure that it is efficacious, effective and efficient.

GLOSSARY OF COMMON TERMS

Birth rate. The number of live births occurring (or occasionally registered) in a year (usually a calendar year) divided by the total mid-year population, expressed as a rate per 1000 of the mid-year population.

Cohort. A cohort is a group of people sharing a common characteristic (such as year of birth).

Death rate. Number of deaths occurring during a specified period of time (usually a calendar year) divided by the total mid-year population and expressed per 1000 of the mid-year population.

Epidemiology. The study of disease in populations.

Evaluation. The attempt to see whether specified objectives have been achieved, and if so to what extent.

Fertility rate. The live births occurring (or occasionally registered) divided by the female population of child bearing age (usually 15-44 years).

Health. 'A state of complete physical, mental and social well-being and not merely the absence of disease or infirmity' (from the Constitution of the World Health Organisation).

Incidence. The number of new cases of disease arising, in a defined population, over a defined period of time.

Perinatal mortality. The number of deaths in the first week of life, plus the number of stillbirths, expressed as a rate per 1000 total births (live and stillbirths) in a defined calendar year.

Prevalence. The proportion of existing cases of a disease in a defined population. *Point prevalence* gives a figure for one moment in time. *Period prevalence* gives a figure for cases existing at any time during a period of time (for example during one year).

Research.   Conscious action to acquire deeper knowledge or new facts about scientific or technical subjects.

Screening.   The application of usually simple tests to generally large numbers of individuals, who do not have specific symptoms, but who attend in the hope of obtaining medical benefit.

Standardised Mortality Ratio (SMR).   The rates of deaths at all ages observed in a given population to the deaths that are expected on the basis of each age (and sex) group being exposed to some selected standard rates.

Stillbirth rates.   The number of stillbirths (intra-uterine deaths after the twenty-eighth week of pregnancy) occurring during one year in every 1000 total births (live and stillbirths).

BIBLIOGRAPHY

Alphey, R.S. and Leach, J.S. (1974) 'Accidental Deaths in the Home', *Royal Society of Health Journal*, 3, 97-102.

Ashton, J.R. (1980) *Everyday Psychiatry*, Update Books, London, pp. 12-16.

Backett, M.E. (1965) *Domestic Accidents*, World Health Organisation, Geneva.

Balke, F.G. and Howell-Wright, F. (1963) *Essentials of Paediatric Nursing*, Pitmans, Kent.

Baly, M.E. (1973) *Nursing and Social Change*, Heinemann, London, p. 61.

Barker, D.J.P. (1982) 'Changing Patterns of Disease in Britain in the Last 50 Years', in *150th Anniversary Issue British Medical Journal*, British Medical Association, London, pp. 18-20.

Barker, D.J.P and Rose, G. (1979) *Epidemiology in Medical Practice*, Churchill Livingstone, Edinburgh, p. 40.

Basu, R.N., Jezek, Z. and Ward, N.A. (1979) *The Eradication of Smallpox from India*, World Health Organisation, New Delhi, pp. 187-223.

Bradford-Hill, A. (1966) 'Principles of Medical Statistics', *Lancet*, London, p. 22.

Breman, J.G. and Arita, I. (1980) 'The Confirmation and Maintenance of Smallpox Eradication', *New England Journal of Medicine*, 303, 1263-73.

Brewer, W. and Rowe R.G. (1972) *Hospital Activity Analysis: An Account of the National Computer Based Information System*, Butterworth, London.

Brockington, C.F. (1965) *The Health of the Community*, J. and A. Churchill, London, pp. 32-3.

Ibid., p. 34.

Ibid., p. 43.

Burgess, C., Chant, A.D.B. and Beschi, J. (1978) 'Elective Surgery and a Programmed Investigation Unit in a Five Day Ward', *Hospital and Health Services Review*, 74, 427-8.

Cargill, D. (1967) *Accidents in the Home*, Hamish Hamilton, London.

Carstairs, V. (1981) 'Our Elders', in R.F.A. Shegog (ed.), *The Impending Crisis of Old Age*, Oxford University Press, Oxford, pp. 31-3.

Cartwright, F.F. (1977) *A Social History of Medicine*, Longman, London, p. 103.

Ibid., pp. 186-7.

Chant, A.D.B., Jones, H.O. and Weddell, J.M. (1972) 'Varicose Veins: A Comparison of Surgery and Infection/Compression Sclerotherapy', *Lancet*, 2, 1188-91.

Clarke, M.G. (1980) 'Psychiatric Liaison with Health Visitors', *Health Trends*, 12, 98-100.

Cliff, K.S. (1973) 'Home Accidents: A Study of Patients attending Hospital Accident and Emergency Departments as a Result of Home Accidents', *Care in the Home*, 5, 4-7.

Cochrane, A.L. (1971) *Effectiveness and Efficiency: Random Reflections on the National Health Service*, Nuffield Provincial Hospital Trust, London.

Community Medicine (1982), 1, 49.

Cooper, B. and Morgan, H.G. (1973) *Epidemiological Psychiatry*, Charles Thomas, Illinois, USA, pp. 20-3.

Davenport, C.D. and Muncey, E.B. (1916) 'Huntington's Chorea in Relation to Heredity and Eugenics', *American Journal of Insanity*, 73, 195-222.

Davies, R., Cliff, K.S. and Waters, W.E. (1981) 'Present Use of Five-Day Wards', *British Medical Journal*, 2, 2118-19.

Dean, K.G. and James, D.H. (1980) 'The Spatial Distribution of Depressive Illness in Plymouth', *British Journal of Psychiatry*, 136, 167-80.

Department of Health and Social Security (1976) *Prevention and Health: Everybody's Business*, HMSO, London.

Department of Health and Social Security (1981) *Prevention and Health: Avoiding Heart Attacks*, HMSO, London.

Department of Prices and Consumer Protection (1976) *Collection of Information on Accidents in the Home*, Department of Prices and Consumer Protection, London, p. 11.

Department of Prices and Consumer Protection (1977) *The Home Accident Surveillance System. Report of the First Six Months' Data Collection*, Department of Prices and Consumer Protection, London, p. 4.

Ibid., p. 7.

Department of Trade (1981) *The 'Home Accident Surveillance System' 1980 — Presentation of Twelve Months' Data (The Fourth Twelve Months)*, Department of Trade, London, pp. 28-31.

Ibid., p. 18.

Department of Transport (1980) *Road Accidents Great Britain 1978*, HMSO, London, pp. xi-xii.

Doll, R. (1955) 'Mortality from Lung Cancer in Asbestos Workers', *British Journal of Industrial Medicine*, 12, 81-6.

Doll, R. and Hill, A.B. (1950) 'Smoking and Carcinoma of the Lung: Preliminary Report', *British Medical Journal*, 2, 739-48.

Doll, R. and Hill, A.B. (1964) 'Mortality in Relation to Smoking: Ten Years' Observations in British Doctors', *British Medical Journal*, 1, 1399-410, 1460-7.

Donnan, S.P.B. and Lambert, P.M. (1976) 'Appendicitis: Incidence and Mortality', *Population Trends*, 5, 26-8.

Essex-Cater, A. (1967) *A Synopsis of Public Health and Social Medicine*, J. Wright and Sons, Bristol, p. 73.

Farrer-Brown, L. and Warren, M.D. (1965) *Public Health and Social Services*, Edward Arnold, London, pp. 94-7.

Frazer, W.M. (1950) *A History of English Public Health 1834-1939*, Baillière Tindall and Cox, London, pp. 229-30.

Ibid., pp. 63-4.

Frerichs, R.R., Aneshensel, C.S. and Clark, A.C. (1981) 'Prevalence of Depression in Los Angeles County', *American Journal of Epidemiology*, 113, 691-9.

Gardner, M.J. (1973) 'Using the Environment to Explain and Predict Mortality', *Journal of the Royal Statistical Society*, 136, 421-40.

Giggs, J. (1973) 'High Rates of Schizophrenia among Immigrants in Nottingham', *Nursing Times*, 2, 1210-12.

Goulding, R. (1975) 'Chemical Hazards in the Home', *British Medical Bulletin*, 31, 191-5.

Green, D.E. (1970) 'Nurses are Kicking the Habit', *American Journal of Nursing*, 70, 1936-8.

Hancock, B.W. (1973) 'Accidental Poisoning in Childhood', *British Journal of Clinical Practice*, 3, 77-80.

Haward, R.A. and Schofield, R. (1978) 'Typhoid: Diagnostic Difficulties and their Implications for Medical Officers for Environmental Health', *Public Health*, London, 92, 181-5.

Hobbs, C.A. (1978) *The Effectiveness of Seat Belts in Reducing Injuries to Car Occupants*, Transport and Road Research Laboratory Report 811, Crowthorne, Berks, pp. 13-14.

Hobbs, C.A. (1981) *Car Occupant Injury Patterns and Mechanisms*, Transport and Road Research Laboratory Supplementary Report 648, Crowthorne, Berks.

Jackson, R.H. (ed.) (1977) *'Children the Environment and Accidents'*, Pitman Medical, Kent.

Joint Working Group of the Royal College of Physicians of London and British Cardiac Society (1976) 'Prevention of Coronary Heart Disease', *Journal of the Royal College of Physicians*, 10, 213-75.

Kash, S.V. and Cobb, S. (1966) 'Health Behaviour, Illness Behaviour and Sick Role Behaviour', *Archives of Environmental Health*, 12, 246-66.

Kilzinger, S. (1979) *The Experience of Breast Feeding*, Croom Helm, London, p. 18.

Knox, E.G. (1979) *Epidemiology in Health Care Planning*, Oxford University Press, Oxford.

Kushlick, A. (1966) 'A Community Service for the Mentally Subnormal', *Social Psychiatry*, 1, 73-82.

Longston, D. and Young, B. (1973) 'The Manchester Royal Infirmary Programmed Investigation Unit', *Briitsh Medical Journal* 4, 528-31.

Lock, S. and Smith, T. (1977) *The Medical Risks of Life*, Penguin Books, Harmondsworth, pp. 42-6.

MacMahon, B. and Pugh, T.F. (1970) *Epidemiology: Principles and Methods*, Little Brown, Boston, USA.

Minear, D. and Lucente, F.E. (1979) 'Current Attitudes of Laryngectomy Patients', *Laryngoscope*, 89, 1061-5.

Morrel, D.C., Gage, H.G. and Robinson, N.A. (1970) 'Patterns of Demand in General Practice', *Journal of the Royal College of General Practitioners*, 19, 331-41.

Morris, D., Ward, A.W.M. and Handyside, A.J. (1968) 'Early Discharge After Hernia Repair', *Lancet*, 1, 681-5.

Moser, C.A. and Kalton, G. (1972) *Survey Methods in Social Investigation*, Heinemann, London, p. 127.

Ibid., pp. 238-377.

McKeown, T. and Lowe, C.R. (1977) *'An Introduction to Social Medicine'*, Blackwell, Oxford, p. 5.

Ibid., pp. 19-20.

Ibid., p. 144.

McMullen, D.K. (1976) 'A Study of Depressive Illness Among Patients in a Group Practice', *Nursing Times*, 72, 504-8.

Newhouse, M.L. (1979) 'The Asbestos Industry and Statutory Control of its Hazards', *International Agency for Research on Cancer: Scientific Publication*, 74, 59-70.

Niel, J.V., Clark, D. and Muller, M. (1980) 'The Smoking Patterns and Attitudes of Student Nurses and Student Teachers', *The Australian Nurses' Journal*, 9, 47-8.

Nielsen, J. and Nielsen, J.A. (1977) 'A Census Study of Mental Illness in Samsø', *Psychological Medicine*, 7, 491-503.

Office of Health Economics (1978) *Renal Failure: A Priority in Health?*, Office of Health Economics No. 62, London.

Office of Health Economics (1979) *Scarce Resources in Health Care*, Office of Health Economics No. 64, London.

Office of Population Censuses and Surveys (1980) *Population and Health Statistics in England and Wales*, Office of Population Censuses and Surveys, London, p. 1.

Ibid., p. 4.

Ibid., p. 24.

Office of Population Censuses and Surveys (1981) *Mortality Statistics Accidents and Violence 1979 (England and Wales)*, HMSO, London, p. 11.

Ibid., pp. 12-24.

Office of Population Censuses and Surveys (1982) *Estimates of Cancer Registrations 1978 (England and Wales)*, HMSO, London, p. 2.

Parry, W.H. (1973) *Communicable Diseases, An Epidemiological Approach*, English Universities Press, London, pp. 156-9.

Pickles, W.N. (1932) 'Sonne Dysentry in Yorkshire Dales', *Lancet*, 2, 31-2.

Raine, D.N. (ed.) (1975) *The Treatment of Inherited Disorders*, Medical and Technical Publishing, Lancaster.

Reeder, S.J., Mastroianni, L. and Martin, L.L. (1980) *Maternity Nursing*, Lippincott Company, Philadelphia, pp. 476-7.

Report of the Royal Commission on Medical Education (1968) (Todd Report) Cmnd 3569, HMSO, London, pp. 66-70.

Roberts, A. (1982) 'Cervical Cytology in England and Wales 1965-1980', *Health Trends*, 2, 41-3.

Roberts, C.J. (1977) *Epidemiology for Clinicians*, Pitman Medical, Kent, pp. 86-9.

Rock, W.P., Gordon, P.H. and Bradnock, G. (1981) 'Dental Caries in Birmingham and Wolverhampton School Children following the Fluoridation of Birmingham Water in 1964', *British Dental Journal*, 3, 61-6.

Rose, G.A. and Blackburn, H. (1968) *Cardiovascular Survey Methods*, World Health Organisation, Geneva.

Seymer, L.R. (1957) *Florence Nightingale*, Faber and Faber, London, pp. 84-5.

Shim, C.S. and Williams, M.H. (1980) 'Evaluation of the Severity of Asthma: Patients versus Physicians', *The American Journal of Medicine*, 68, 11-13.

Singer, C. (1928) *A Short History of Medicine*, Clarendon Press, London, pp. 78-80.

Small, W.P. and Tucker, L. (1978) 'The Smoking Habits of Hospital Nurses', *Nursing Times*, 2, 1878-9.

Smith, C. (1976) 'Accidents in the Elderly', *Nursing Times*, 2, 1872-6.

Smith, T. (1982) 'The Wasted Years', *Nursing Mirror*, 154, 17.

Social Trends (1980) 10, 90.

Social Trends (1982) 12, 128.

Tunstall Pedoe, H. (1982) 'Coronary Heart Disease', in D.L. Miller and R.D.T. Farmer (eds.), *Epidemiology of Disease*, Blackwell, Oxford.

University of Southampton Community Medicine (1982) *Home Accidents in Children under Five (Fourth Year Student Project)*, Community Medicine, Southampton.

Watts, C.A.H. (1966) *Depressive Disorders in the Community*, John Wright and Sons, Bristol, pp. 30-3.

Wessex Positive Health Team (1980) *Promoting the Use of Seat Belts in Wessex*, Wessex Regional Health Authority, Winchester.

Wessex Regional Hospital Board (1973) *Report on the Accident and Emergency Services*, Wessex Regional Hospital Board, Winchester.

West, R.R., Crosby, D.L. and Jones, J.H. (1974) 'Mathematical Model of an Integrated Haemodialysis and Renal Transplantation Programme', *British Journal of Preventive and Social Medicine*, 28, 149-55.

Whitwell, F., Scott, J. and Grimshaw, M. (1977) 'Relationship Between Occupation and Asbestos Fibre Content of the Lung in Patients with Pleural Mesothelioma, Lung Cancer and other Diseases', *Thorax*, 32, 377-86.

Wigfield, W.J. (1976) 'Cancer Screening in East Sussex', *Public Health*, 90, 65-73.

Wilkie, E. (1979) *The History of the Council for the Education and Training of Health Visitors*, Allen and Unwin, London.

World Health Organisation (1978) *Manual of the International Statistical Classification of Diseases, Injuries and Causes of Death, Vol. 1*, World Health Organisation, Geneva.

INDEX